LIMITED RADIOGRAPHY

DEDICATION

To my loving mothor Faye
who is my best friend and supporter

My grandparents Kat and Joe,
my family, Rick, Sloan, and Jennifer,
to Lee, Louise and all those
who believe in me

A great thanks to all who provided support
and encouragement for a woman to pursue "her dream."

LIMITED RADIOGRAPHY

Frances Campeau
Jeana Phelps

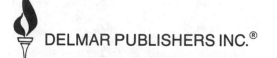DELMAR PUBLISHERS INC.®

NOTICE TO THE READER

Cover Design by: Carol L. Cornette

Delmar Staff
  Executive Editor: David Gordon
  Associate Editor: Marion Waldman
  Developmental Editor: Marjorie A. Bruce
  Project Editor: Carol Micheli
  Production Supervisor: Larry Main
  Art Coordinator: John Lent
  Design Coordinator: Karen Kemp

Delmar Publishers' Online Services
To access Delmar on the World Wide Web, point your browser to:
http://www.delmar.com/delmar.html
To access through Gopher: gopher://gopher.delmar.com
(Delmar Online is part of "thomson.com", an Internet site with information on more than 30 publishers of the International Thomson Publishing organization.)
For information on our products and services:
email: info@delmar.com
or call 800-347-7707

For information, address Delmar Publishers Inc.
3 Columbia Circle
Albany, New York 12212

COPYRIGHT © 1993
BY DELMAR PUBLISHERS INC.

Printed in the United States of America
Published simultaneously in Canada
by Nelson Canada,
a division of The Thomson Corporation

10 9 8 7 6

Library of Congress Cataloging-in-Publication Data
Campeau, Frances.
  Limited radiography / Frances Campeau, Jeana Phelps.
    p. cm.
  Includes index.
  ISBN 0-8273-3335-8
  1. Radiography, Medical. 2. Radiography, Medical — Vocational
guidance. I. Phelps, Jeana. II. Title.
  [DNLM: 1. Radiography. WN 200 C193L]
RC78.C33   1992
616.07'572 — dc20
DNLM/DLC
for Library of Congress
                                                    92-49682
                                                    CIP

Contents

Index of Tables

Preface

The radiography professions have seen many changes since Congress passed the Consumer-Patient Radiation Health and Safety Act (Public Law 97-35). The Act requires the Secretary of Health and Human Services to develop minimum standards for state accreditation of radiologic technology education programs and state certification or licensure of persons who administer ionizing and/or nonionizing radiation in medical and dental radiologic procedures.

For many years, the radiologic technologist was the only level of worker who was tested and credentialed. The radiologic technologist completed a two-year program approved by the Committee on Allied Health Education Accreditation (CAHEA). As a result of Public Law 97-35, many states have adopted education and certification standards for radiation workers other than the two-year radiographers. The Limited Permittee, as these other workers are often known, are usually employed in physicians' offices, chiropractic and dental clinics, and in ambulatory care settings.

In 1985, the American Registry of Radiologic Technologists (ARRT) identified a task listing and began development of an examination that can be used by states that license limited permittees. The ARRT indicates that the depth of required knowledge is the same for all radiographers; it is the scope of practice that differentiates the levels of radiographers.

The goal of this text is to meet the needs of the radiographer in limited practice and to upgrade the performance standards in these areas of practice. The authors have designed the text for students at the post-secondary level who plan to test for certification in limited radiography. It is also an excellent reference for medical workers who are participating in independent self-study programs for limited radiography.

The goal of the text is to provide students with a fundamental imaging foundation so that they are competent clinical practitioners capable of producing diagnostic radiographs while subjecting the patient and health care personnel to minimum radiation exposure.

The first three chapters introduce the student to radiography as a career. Topics covered include educational requirements, continuing education, professionalism, professional relationships, concepts for effective communication, and law and ethics specific to limited radiography.

Chapter 4 is concerned with medical aspects and patient care. The principles of infection control and universal precautions are stressed for the safety of the patient and health care workers. Basic concepts of patient care, including safety considerations and moving and transporting are also discussed.

Chapter 5 presents the basic concepts of radiation physics, beginning with the theory of atomic structure and continuing through the principles of electricity and magnetism. These concepts are then applied in chapters 6–9, which are concerned with the technical aspects of radiography: production of radiation, imaging equipment, film exposure and film processing. Chapter 10 covers the evaluation of radiographic film images.

Chapters 11 and 12 are concerned with the safety of ionizing radiation. Chapter 11 covers the effect of ionizing radiation on human cells and tissues while chapter 12 discusses radiation protection procedures and radiation detection and monitoring.

In selected chapters reference is made to specific tasks for which students of limited radiography must demonstrate competence. These tasks are outlined in the appendix. For each task, the following information is given: procedural title, terminal performance objective, a listing of equipment and supplies, and a performance guide (numbered sequential steps from the beginning to the end of the task).

The text does not discuss radiographic anatomy and positioning since there are many excellent texts available that deal in detail with these areas. The authors believe that by not "reinventing the wheel" they have been able to focus on the didactic presentation of radiographic imaging and radiation protection.

An Instructor's Guide accompanies the text. The guide includes answers to the chapter reviews and competency checklists for the procedural tasks listed in the text appendix.

Frances E. Campeau, MA, RT(R)
Jeana Phelps, MEd, RT

Acknowledgments

The idea for a textbook devoted to limited radiography has been in the minds of the authors for many years, long before its need became apparent. Planning a book and actually writing are two separate functions and the reality of bringing this book to fruition would not have been possible without certain other people.

We are forever indebted to Ms. Nancy C. Roubieu, whose enduring patience was responsible for the production of the manuscript and who was an indispensable editor.

Dr. A. Michael Connor also added his expertise in assisting with the critical revision of several chapters to make substantive information more salient.

Ms. Sophia Fleming has been a valuable adjunct in many ways, helping to meet deadlines (when they were met), running errands, typing all the correspondence to the publisher, taking messages, and generally providing liaison among all concerned parties. Our friends and colleagues also have been supportive with ideas and just listening when it was needed.

Frances E. Campeau, MA, RT(R)
Jeana Phelps, MEd, RT

* * * * * * * * *

The Delmar staff wishes to thank the professionals who reviewed the manuscript in its several stages. Appreciation for their constructive recommendations is extended to:

Fred Goodwin, RT (ARRT), CRT, Long Beach City College, Long Beach, CA 90808

Sandra L. Kerr, BSRT(R), Radiation Physicist, Bureau of Radiological Health, Department of Environmental Protection, State of New Jersey, Trenton, NJ 08625-0415

Shelley Matzen, University of Iowa, Iowa City, IA 52242

Mary G. DiStefano, Bureau of Radiological Health, Department of Environmental Protection, State of New Jersey, Trenton, NJ 08625-0415

Sharon A. Coffey, RT, Houston Community College, Houston, TX 77021

Denise Vill'Neuve, RT, BS, Bergen Community College, Paramus, NJ 07652

Lynn Rhatigan, BS, RT, Berdan Institute, Totowa, NJ 07512

Nancy Johnson, RT(R), Tempe Technical Institute, Phoenix, AZ 85004

Francine J. Knutson, BEd, RT(R), Educational Foundation, Inc. of the American Society of Radiological Technologists, Albuquerque, NM 87123

Louise Kay Kavanagh, MSRT(R), Indiana Vocational Technical College, Indianapolis, IN 46206

Sarah Baker, MS, RT(R), Indiana University School of Medicine, Indianapolis, IN 46223

Helen L. Cook, RT(R), Southeastern Community College, Mount Pleasant, IA 52641

* * * * * * * *

The following companies provided technical information, illustrations and/or photographs.

Eastman Kodak Company

General Electric Medical Systems

IVAC Corporation

CHAPTER

1

Introduction to Limited Radiography: The Occupation

CHAPTER OUTLINE

Introduction
History, Purpose, and Functions
    Philosophy Statement
    Occupational Scope and Purpose
Education
Continuing Education and Professional Organizations
Occupational Progress and Professionalization
The Future

OBJECTIVES

Upon completion of the chapter, the student will meet the following objectives by verifying knowledge of the facts and principles presented through oral and written communication at a level deemed competent.

1. Identify the occupational role and function of the limited radiographer.
2. Describe the impact of the Consumer-Patient Radiation Health and Safety Act on the development of the limited radiography occupation.
3. Discuss the role of continuing education in the professional growth and development of a limited radiographer.
4. List several prospects for employment as a limited radiographer.

INTRODUCTION

Does the term **limited radiography** designate a new occupation emerging within the radiological sciences, or does it designate a skill level within the radiological sciences consisting of limited radiography tasks performed by a myriad of workers in medical offices, clinics, and ambulatory care centers?

Why are individuals who operate radiation-producing equipment coming under state and federal guidelines and regulations that address the establishment of minimum educational standards, competency testing, and continuing education? Who are limited radiographers, how are they educated, and where are they employed? Do limited radiographers and radiologic technologists share a common professional role but differ in their level of responsibility and scope of practice? These are just a few of the many questions being asked today about limited radiography and individuals called limited radiographers. This chapter will focus on the essential characteristics of limited radiography as an occupation.

HISTORY, PURPOSE, AND FUNCTIONS

On November 8, 1895, Wilhelm Conrad Roentgen announced his discovery of a new kind of radiant energy. Investigating conduction of electrons through a partially evacuated glass tube, he found that a plate coated with a fluorescent material emitted light when struck by rays from the glass tube. Using the nomenclature for the algebraic unknown ("X"), Roentgen called the mysterious new light "X ray." In the early years, Roentgen and others used X rays to diagnose bone fractures, examine internal organs, and locate foreign objects in tissues. Today, because of scientific advancements in equipment design, *radiology*—a branch of medical science that uses radiant energies—has a far wider scope of application and includes many areas of specialization, such as radiation therapy, nuclear medicine, ultrasound, special procedures, and computed tomography. Figure 1-1 is an overview of areas of specialization in the field of radiography.

Although diversity and specialization exist within the radiological sciences, a core of knowledge and skills is common to all radiographers. Beyond this basic core, there are distinct differences between the scope of practice of a limited radiographer and a radiologic technologist. The differences (educational and scope of practice) between a radiologic technologist and a limited radiographer are readily apparent in the following descriptions.

A *radiologic technologist* has successfully completed a formal educational program evaluated by the Joint Review Committee on Education in

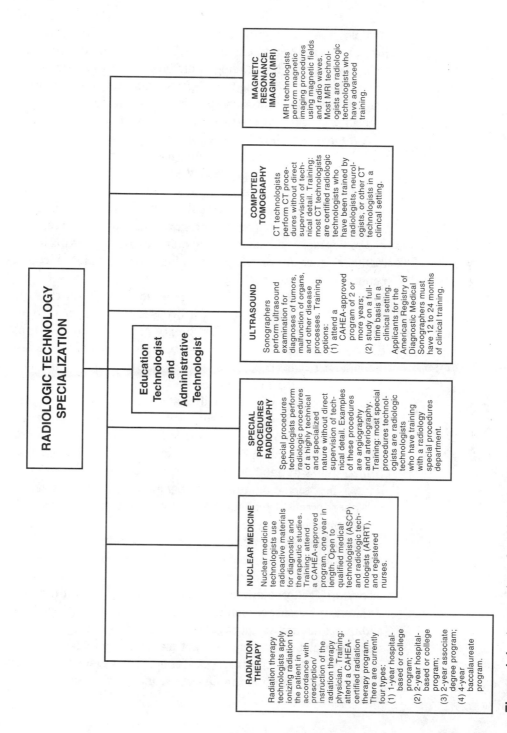

RADIOLOGIC TECHNOLOGY SPECIALIZATION

Education Technologist and Administrative Technologist

RADIATION THERAPY

Radiation therapy technologists apply ionizing radiation to the patient in accordance with prescription/instruction of the radiation therapy physician. Training: attend a CAHEA-certified radiation therapy program. There are currently four types:
(1) 1-year hospital-based or college program;
(2) 2-year hospital-based or college program;
(3) 2-year associate degree program;
(4) 4-year baccalaureate program.

NUCLEAR MEDICINE

Nuclear medicine technologists use radioactive materials for diagnostic and therapeutic studies. Training: attend a CAHEA-approved program, one year in length. Open to qualified medical technologists (ASCP) and radiologic technologists (ARRT), and registered nurses.

SPECIAL PROCEDURES RADIOGRAPHY

Special procedures technologists perform radiologic procedures of a highly technical and specialized nature without direct supervision of technical detail. Examples of these procedures are angiography and arteriography. Training: most special procedures technologists are radiologic technologists who have training with a radiology special procedures department.

ULTRASOUND

Sonographers perform ultrasound examination for diagnoses of tumors, malfunction of organs, and other disease processes. Training options:
(1) attend a CAHEA-approved program of 2 or more years;
(2) study on a full-time basis in a clinical setting. Applicants for the American Registry of Diagnostic Medical Sonographers must have 12 to 24 months of clinical training.

COMPUTED TOMOGRAPHY

CT technologists perform CT procedures without direct supervision of technical detail. Training: most CT technologists are certified radiologic technologists who have been trained by radiologists, neurologists, or other CT technologists in a clinical setting.

MAGNETIC RESONANCE IMAGING (MRI)

MRI technologists perform magnetic imaging procedures using magnetic fields and radio waves. Most MRI technologists are radiologic technologists who have advanced training.

Figure 1-1. An overview of specialization in Radiologic Technology

Radiologic Technology and approved by the Committee on Allied Health Education and Accreditation (CAHEA). Radiologic technologists perform both basic and contrast radiographic procedures as supervised by a licensed practitioner of the healing arts (a person licensed or otherwise authorized to practice medicine, dentistry, podiatry, osteopathy, or chiropractic). These procedures may be performed in hospitals or other medical care settings.

A *limited radiographer* may have completed formal allied health education in a program such as nursing, medical assisting, medical technology, respiratory therapy, or physical therapy. Such programs generally do not provide radiography education; however, cross training, or a multiskilled approach, is common in medical assisting programs. Individuals coming from allied health educational programs who have not received formal limited radiography education may acquire radiography skills by less traditional methods, such as on-the-job training, correspondence courses, or independent study programs.

A limited radiographer performs basic noncontrast radiographic procedures under the supervision of a licensed practitioner of the healing arts. Limited radiographers generally do not perform specialized radiography or fluoroscopic procedures. These procedures often include the use of contrast media and require specific education and training beyond the scope of the duties of a limited radiographer.

Limited radiographers usually are employed in medical offices and outpatient and ambulatory care clinics; in some states, they are also employed in hospitals. A variety of occupational titles exists for workers/staff who perform limited radiography tasks; such titles vary from one area of the United States to another. Thus, the limited radiographer may be called a limited license radiographer, radiographic assistant, limited medical radiographer, practical technologist, or, most recently, limited permittee.

Radiographers may be further classified by state laws that regulate the scope of practice. A number of states recognize ten specific Limited Permittee categories for radiographers: chest, extremities, gastrointestinal, skull, torso-skeletal, dermatology, genito-urinary, leg and podiatric, dental laboratory, and photofluorographic chest. Table 1-1 illustrates geographic differences in occupational titles and regulations. If the reader should desire additional information about classification of radiographers and radiographic tasks in a particular state, contact that state's Radiation Control Office. A listing of such offices may be obtained by contacting The Conference of Radiation Control Program Directors, Inc., 205 Capital Avenue, Frankfort, Kentucky 40601.

TABLE 1-1 LIMITED MEDICAL RADIOGRAPHY LICENSURE INFORMATIONAL MATRIX

STATE	LICENSURE BEGAN	CATEGORIES FOR LIMITED RADIOGRAPHY
Arizona	1978	(3) Practical Technologist; Practical Technologist in Radiology (Chest for lung visualization and Extremities limited to lower two-thirds of humerus and lower distal one-third of femur); Practical Technologist in Podiatry (limited to lower leg below knee). No mandatory CEUs.*
California	1971	(10) Limited Permittee: Chest, Extremities, G.I., Skull, Torso-Skeletal, Dermatology, G.U., Leg and Podiatric, Dental Lab, Photofluorographic Chest. California requires twenty-five hours of CEUs every five years. CEU standards in place.
Delaware	1987	(1) Radiation Technologist: Any individual who is a dental auxiliary or medical radiographer.
Florida	1979	(1) Basic X-ray Machine Operator. Requires twelve hours of continuing education every two years.
Illinois	1984	(3) Medical Radiography, Pediatric Radiographic Assistant, Chiropractic Radiographic Assistant. Requires twelve hours every year. CEU standards in place.
Indiana	1981	(5) Limited Certification: Chest, Podiatry, Dental, Chiropractic, Limited General. No mandatory CEUs.
Iowa	1983	Limited Diagnostic Radiographer (Podiatric, Vertebral Spines, Chest, Extremities and Hospital Limited). Requires twelve hours of CEUs every two years. CEU standards in place.
Kentucky	1978	Limited Medical Radiographer (General Medical). Limited certificate requires twelve hours of CEUs every two years. General certificate requires eighteen hours of CEUs every two years.
Louisiana	1984	Chiropractic Assistants and assistants in private medical offices/clinics seek authorization. CEU standards in place.
Maine	1984	(6) Limited Radiographer: Trunk, Spine and Innominate, Chest, Extremities, Leg and Foot, Skull. No mandatory CEUs in place.
Maryland	1986	Limited Radiography. Requires thirty hours of CEUs every two years. CEU standards or requirements.
Massachusetts	1988	Category regulations have not yet been promulgated. No mandatory CEU standards or requirements.

*CEU = continuing education unit

TABLE 1-1 (CONT'D)

STATE	LICENSURE BEGAN	CATEGORIES FOR LIMITED RADIOGRAPHY
Minnesota		The Minnesota Department of Health is authorized to license allied health personnel but has not promulgated regulations.
Montana	1977	(5) Limited Permit: Chest, Extremities, Spine, Skull, other including Fluoroscopy. No mandatory CEU requirements.
New Jersey	1969	(5) Licensed X-ray Technologist: Chest, Podiatric, Dental, Urologic, Orthopedic. No mandatory CEU requirements, but standards in place.
New Mexico	1983	Limited Radiologic Practitioner. Requires twenty hours of CEUs every two years.
Oregon	1979	(6) Limited Permit: Skull and Sinuses, Spine, Chest and Ribs, Upper Extremities, Lower Extremities, Abdomen and Pelvis. Requires twelve hours of CEUs every year. CEU standards in place.
Pennsylvania	1987	The Department of State is authorized to license operators of X-ray equipment but has not promulgated regulations.
South Carolina	1986	Specific regulations have not yet been promulgated.
Tennessee	1982	(2) Certified X-ray Operator: Chest and Extremity Radiography. No mandatory CEU requirements or standards.
Texas	1988	Limited Certificate: Chest, Extremities, Spine, Dental, Chiropractic, Podiatric, and Skull. Limited Medical Radiologic Technologist (LMRT). General Certificate: Medical Radiologic Technologist (MRT).
Vermont	1978	(3) Limited Radiography License: Chest, Extremities, Chest and Extremities. No mandatory CEUs required.
West Virginia	1978	Limited Permit: certification regulations pending. No mandatory CEU requirements. CEU standards identified and in place.
Wyoming	1985	Radiologic Technician: Person who has not received formal training but who meets minimum requirements for restricted license. Requires five hours of CEUs every year. No standards in place.

Note: Hawaii and New York have identified CEU standards for limited radiographers but have not set minimum requirements.

In 1981, Public Law 97-35 (the Consumer-Patient Radiation Health and Safety Act) was enacted in response to growing concern and awareness about potential long-term effects from radiation exposure.[1] The act gave Congress the power to protect consumers and patients from unnecessary or excessive radiation exposure. To do so, Congress established the following objectives.

1. Provide for the establishment of minimum standards by the federal government for the accreditation of education programs for persons who administer radiologic procedures and for certification of such persons.
2. Ensure that medical and dental radiologic procedures are consistent with rigorous safety precautions and standards.

On 11 December 1985 in the *Federal Register*, the Secretary of Health and Human Services issued 42 CFR Part 75—minimum Standards for Accreditation of Educational Programs For, and the Credentialing of Radiologic Personnel; Final Rule.[2] These standards are intended for use by states in implementing Public Law 97-35.

As of 1989–1990, twenty-six states had complied with or were in the process of complying with the 1981 Consumer-Patient Radiation Safety Act. No sanctions have thus far been imposed upon states that choose to ignore the standards. Refer again to Table 1-1 for an overview of the states that have licensure or certification of limited radiographers.

Philosophy Statement

In its relation to a health care profession, a philosophy statement speaks to the motivating concepts or principles guiding the practice of that profession. Thus, the following philosophy statement of the scope of practice for limited radiography attempts to capture the intent of the Consumer-Patient Radiation Health and Safety Act.

A limited radiographer is a multiskilled person dedicated to assisting in many aspects of medical care. These duties are at the request of and under the supervision of a licensed practitioner of the healing arts. The limited radiographer's scope of practice is confined to radiography of anatomic parts and body regions as regulated by applicable state laws. Although their scope of practice may be confined by law, limited radiographers must have the depth of knowledge and understanding necessary for each radiographic task to assure skill competency and safety as a practitioner. Competence in the occupation also requires that a limited radiographer demonstrate professional characteristics, adhere to ethical and legal standards of medical practice, communicate effectively, and recognize and respond to emergencies to provide maximum protection to the patient.

Occupational Scope and Purpose

Job requirements and responsibilities of a limited radiographer vary from office to office or other practice site; particular qualifications and responsibilities depend upon the medical specialty or geographic area of employment. The scope of duties limited radiographers perform also depends upon applicable state laws. Regardless of these differences, a basic core of knowledge and skills includes the following broad job duty areas:

1. Communication
2. Administrative and clerical functions
3. Patient care and management
4. Support service duties
5. Operation and maintenance of radiographic imaging equipment
6. Operation and maintenance of film processing equipment and supplies
7. Radiation protection
8. Radiographic imaging and patient positioning
9. Radiographic exposure and quality
10. Continuing education

The more experienced limited radiographer may become an office or clinic manager, supervising other personnel and coordinating the overall operations of a medical practice.

Basic to the occupation is the ability and desire to perform as a cooperative member of a medical team. A good perspective from which to view the occupation is to think of it as being "service oriented" rather than "task oriented." The purpose is to function as a medical team member and to help provide quality care for the person undergoing radiographic procedures.

EDUCATION

During the years when limited radiography was beginning to develop as a distinguishable job category, it was a common practice for allied health workers to learn radiography on the job. Of course, some of these individuals had completed formal educational programs in related fields, such as in nursing, medical technology, or medical assisting; however, most of these workers trained in other fields did not have prior education in radiography per se and learned radiographic procedures on the job.

A number of factors, such as consumer awareness of the dangers of radiation and state compliance with the Consumer-Patient Radiation Health and Safety Act, have resulted in the limited radiographer's occupation becoming more than just a series of tasks that can be taught in an on-the-job learning situation. Rather, a structured competency-based educational system is needed to assure that the limited radiographer is a skilled and safe practitioner. A minimum task list is provided in the publication *Task Inventory for Radiography*, available from The American Registry of Radiologic Technologists, 1255 Northland Drive, Mendota Heights, MN 55120.

Many states have adopted the Standards for the Accreditation of Educational Programs for, and the Credentialing of Radiologic Personnel provided by the Department of Health and Human Services, 42 CFR Part 75; December 1985. Implementation of limited radiography training varies from state to state. Some states have developed essentials and guidelines for formal limited radiography educational programs and alternatives—for example, correspondence or independent study programs combined with a supervised on-the-job clinical practicum. In 1987, the Joint Review Committee on Education in Radiologic Technology (JRCERT) "announced that it was studying the question whether a mechanism should be created whereby limited scope of practice educational programs could request evaluation by the JRCERT. The type of recognition that would be awarded is being considered."[3] For further information on the status of the educational standards for a particular state, refer again to Table 1-1.

Limited radiography education may be included with other health occupational programs, such as medical assistant or laboratory technician. Some states have limited radiography education programs designed to admit such individuals as registered nurses or licensed practical or vocational nurses, laboratory technologists, chiropractic or medical assistants, physician assistants, or paramedics. The U.S. Department of Education health occupations newsletter *Lines* (Fall edition 1987) reported that "Several states are planning and implementing programs involving multi-competencies. In Oklahoma, two combinations are being considered (1) combining medical assisting...medical laboratory, and radiography and (2) combining radiography, radiation therapy, and sonography."

Figure 1-2 illustrates the cooperation and cross-discipline education occurring between radiology and other allied health professions. The Iowa Administrative Code, Public Health Department [641], rule 42.1 (136 C)

Licensed practical and registered nurses are permitted to practice as diagnostic radiographers while under the supervision of a licensed practitioner, provided that the appropriate training standards for use of radiation emitting equipment are met as outlined in the Iowa Administrative Code, Public Health Department [641], rule 42.1 (136 C).

The rules state that the radiation operator must successfully complete an approved 100-hour limited radiography course, such as those offered by the community colleges or the University of Osteopathic Medicine, or a 2-year general radiography curriculum. Upon completion of the course, the nurse must apply for a permit to perform diagnostic radiography from the Iowa Department of Public Health, (515) 281-3478. Within 1 year of completing the course the licensee must pass the state examination for diagnostic radiography.

Radiography continuing education is approved by the Department of Public Health. The continuing education requirements are 12 contact hours per 2 year period for limited radiographers and 24 contact hours per 2 year period for general radiographers.

Either the basic 100-hour limited radiographer course or continuing education may be used for nursing continuing education *IF* the course is also covered by an Iowa Board of Nursing Provider Number. (Ask the providing institution if the course is covered for nurses.)

Any nurse found to be using radiation emitting equipment who has not met the appropriate training standards shall be subject to appropriate proceedings being initiated by the board to determine if probable cause exists for license revocation, suspension, or probation.

Note. Excerpt from *Nursing Newsletter*, Iowa Board of Nursing, 1223 East Court Avenue, Des Moines, IA 50319, November, December 1987, January 1988.

Figure 1-2. Example of cross-discipline education

states that "licensed practical and registered nurses are permitted to practice as diagnostic radiographers provided they obtain the appropriate training."

The Iowa State Board of Nursing also provides for license revocation, suspension, or probation if any nurse is found to be operating radiation equipment without meeting the appropriate training standards.

The American Registry of Radiologic Technologists (ARRT), founded in 1922, has as its purpose the study and elevation of standards of radiologic technology as well as the examining and certifying of eligible candidates. The ARRT recognizes the following disciplines of radiology certification: radiography, nuclear medicine technology, and radiation therapy technology. As of June 1985, the ARRT began to consider the following areas for advanced level examinations: computer imaging, angiography, and magnetic resonance imaging.

In 1983, at the request of several state licensing agencies, the Board of Trustees of the ARRT began to consider the development of examinations covering the tasks performed by an individual having a scope of practice limited to radiography of the chest and/or extremities. The intended purpose of such examinations was for use by licensing states and not for certification by the ARRT.

The first form of the ARRT Examination for Limited Scope of Practice in Radiography (chest/extremities) was administered on 20 March 1986. Not all licensing states have adopted the ARRT examination; several licensing states administer an examination developed by an advisory group of radiologic technology educators. For further information, contact the American Registry of Radiologic Technologists at 1255 Northland Drive, Mendota Heights, Minnesota 55120.

CONTINUING EDUCATION AND PROFESSIONAL ORGANIZATIONS

Continuing education is encouraged for all allied health professionals and may be obtained by attending professional meetings, seminars, and conventions at county, state, regional, and national levels. Some states have mandatory continuing education policies and require that radiographers show evidence of a certain number of continuing education units (CEUs) in order to renew a certificate or license. Figure 1-3 shows the continuing education sign-in report form used in Kentucky by providers of continuing education units to verify participant attendance.

Continuing education is aimed at improving the quality of work performed by radiographers and increasing their value to the employer and to

SEND TO:
Radiation Operator
  Certification Program
Radiation Control Branch
Bureau for Health Services
275 East Main Street
Frankfort, KY 40601

CONTINUING EDUCATION REPORT FORM
HUMAN RESOURCES/HEALTH SERVICES/RADIATION CONTROL BRANCH
RADIATION OPERATOR CERTIFICATION PROGRAM

NAME	CERTIFICATION NUMBER	SUBJECT TITLE	INSTRUCTOR NAME & TITLE	DATE(S)	HOURS OF INSTRUCTION

Figure 1-3. Kentucky continuing education sign-in report form (adaptation)

everyone seeking medical attention. In addition, by taking part in a professional organization, radiographers have an opportunity to develop valuable job networks, enhance technical knowledge and skills, and have a feeling of professional fellowship within the whole occupation of radiology.

Professional growth often results from experiences encountered in the day-to-day medical arena; however, by participating in an organized radiography association, members make a conscious decision about professional growth. The American Society of Radiologic Technologists (ASRT) was established in 1926 and has affiliate societies in each of the fifty states and the Commonwealth of Puerto Rico as well as district groups within the state societies. The ASRT state and district groups provide regular opportunities for radiographers to meet, network and share ideas, hear speakers, and obtain current medical and scientific information.

The national society and some state affiliates publish journals containing timely information for radiographers. Membership in these groups provides continuing education, professional growth, and an opportunity to develop leadership skills. For additional information about the ASRT affiliate in a particular state, contact the national office (American Society of Radiologic Technologists, 15000 Central Avenue, Albuquerque, NM 87123-4605).

OCCUPATIONAL PROGRESS AND PROFESSIONALIZATION

Since 1981, significant progress has been made toward credentialing operators of ionizing radiation equipment and establishing guidelines for educational programs. However, the next decade will determine if limited radiography will be accepted as a vital and necessary level of practice across the United States.

A new profession within radiology may be emerging; the ingredients certainly exist. The following events are signs that professionalization of limited radiography may soon occur:

- The 1981 Consumer-Patient Radiation Health and Safety Act has set forth mandates for training and credentialing.
- The scope and practice of limited radiography has been defined by many states. A task inventory outlining the scope of practice for limited radiographers has been developed by the American Registry of Radiologic Technologists (ARRT).
- Educational training programs have been developed in many states.
- Continuing education is encouraged and required by some states.

These manifestations reflect professional outlook and behavior.

THE FUTURE

It is a certainty that the demand for radiographers will grow in the future. There is also the possibility that the limited radiography scope of practice will increase as the radiologic technologist is called upon to conduct new procedures using sophisticated imaging modalities. As limited radiographers become better educated and more capable, medical professionals may see an opportunity to utilize a multiskilled person.

The future may also bring professional recognition and full acceptance by established radiography associations, accreditation agencies, and other allied health professions. Another future option includes geographic employment flexibility as more states adopt reciprocity guidelines for licensed or certified limited radiographers. Career advancement and mobility are also future possibilities as career ladders, articulation agreements, and competency challenge examinations are developed to allow limited radiographers to advance into radiologic technology and specialized radiography areas.

REVIEW QUESTIONS

1. In a paragraph, describe and discuss the scope and function of a limited radiographer.
2. Compare and contrast the role and function of a limited radiographer to a radiologic technologist.
3. Name the public law that helped to promote educational standards for limited radiographers.
4. List two major objectives of Public Law 97-35, Consumer-Patient Radiation Safety Act.
5. In a paragraph, explain and discuss the importance of lifelong continuing education and professional development for limited radiographers.

REFERENCES

1. Public Law 97-35. Consumer-Patient Radiation Safety Act. Department of Health and Human Services, Public Health Service.
2. 42 CFR Part 75. Standards for the Accreditation of Educational Programs for, and the Credentialing of Radiologic Personnel; Final Rule. *Federal Register*. Vol 50, No. 238, Wednesday, December 11, 1985. Rules and Regulations, 50710-50724. Part II. Department of Health and Human Services, Public Health Service.
3. The American Registry of Radiologic Technologists. *Annual Report*. Minneapolis, MN: The American Registry of Radiologic Technologists, 1987.

CHAPTER

2

Occupational Standards: Relationships and Communication

CHAPTER OUTLINE

OBJECTIVES

Upon completion of the chapter, the student will meet the following objectives by verifying knowledge of the facts and principles presented through oral and written communication at a level deemed competent.

1. Describe in a written paragraph the importance of positive interpersonal relationships in health care settings.
2. Discuss why there may be differences between how symptomatic and asymptomatic patients perceive the medical environment and suggest ways to avoid miscommunication as a result of these differences.

3. Explain how Abraham Maslow's hierarchy of human needs relates to the radiographer.
4. List three suggestions for creating positive interactions with patients.
5. List and explain five negative barriers to establishing positive relationships.
6. List three suggestions for improving relationships with coworkers, doctors, and supervisors.
7. Describe what is meant by "chain of command" and discuss how it promotes effective communication and team efforts.
8. List five ways the radiographer uses communication in the health care setting.
9. Recall and state an appropriate method of introducing yourself to others.
10. Given sample verbal messages; change them into "I" messages.
11. List five important tips for communicating with referring physicians and agencies.
12. Given sample patient questions, concerns, or statements; use paraphrasing techniques to form a written response.
13. Identify five keys to becoming an effective listener.
14. List five barriers to communication and give suggestions on how to overcome them.
15. Demonstrate competence in each task listed. Refer to the appendix for the individual procedure/performance guides.
    TASKS (See appendix):

    2-1 Using "I" Messages
    2-2 Using Paraphrasing
    2-3 Using Listening Techniques
    2-4 Recognizing Barriers to Communication

Part I: Relationships

INTRODUCTION

Positive interpersonal relationships are established on a foundation of effective communication, both verbal and nonverbal. This chapter presents suggestions and guidelines for establishing positive relationships with others through effective communication. These guidelines are not intended to be an intimidating list of do's and don'ts, nor are they all inclusive. Rather, they are intended to provide practical suggestions about occupational standards of interpersonal relationships and how to relate to others in health care settings. The limited radiographer should consider these suggestions as only a "starting point," then change and adapt them as needed to specific work situations.

INTERPERSONAL RELATIONSHIPS IN HEALTH CARE SETTINGS

Health care is service oriented and requires constant interaction and communication with others. A limited radiographer's typical day involves talking with patients and their families, doctors, other medical personnel, and people in outside agencies and businesses. One must be able to interact and communicate with a variety of personalities and also be able to observe and listen in order to interpret verbal and nonverbal messages.

Recognizing and responding to the needs of others is a first priority for establishing positive relationships. If the limited radiographer, as well as other members of the health care team, adopts a policy of consumer satisfaction as a daily responsibility, everyone who has contact with the medical facility should have a positive image of the medical facility and staff. In the medical environment, professional image is reflected through individual and group behavior. In today's fast-paced medical setting, one may wonder if projecting a positive image and achieving consumer satisfaction are attainable on a daily basis? Why are these goals a challenge in health care settings? One explanation may be that the nature of the health care environment itself creates a stressful, demanding situation that poses threats and fosters fears, anxieties, and apprehensions.

Interpersonal Relationships with Patients

Limited radiographers generally serve two classifications of patients: those who are not ill or do not have any disease symptoms (*asymptomatic* patients) and those who exhibit disease symptoms (*symptomatic* patients). Asymptomatic patients may be in the medical facility to undergo a routine diagnostic examination. These patients may react and communicate differently from patients who are symptomatic and experiencing pain or discomfort. Differences between patients and their reasons for seeking medical care are key elements in the way patients perceive the medical environment. Most people will have some anxiety, apprehension, and fear of the unknown, yet the degree to which individuals experience these feelings is closely linked to their reason(s) for being a patient. Try to recall or imagine your personal feelings in the following situations:

- You are a patient for an annual checkup. You are in excellent physical condition and feel healthy.
- You are a patient for an examination. You have found a lump in your right breast during self-examination.
- You have smoked one pack of cigarettes every day since you were fourteen years old and have suddenly developed a cough.

The relationship of needs, perceptions, and behaviors can be further explained by considering the hierarchy of human needs.

Hierarchy of Human Needs.   All humans have needs that must be met for both physiological and psychological survival and growth. Physiological needs are related to survival (food, water, air, shelter), whereas psychological needs relate to requirements for love, belonging, and self-esteem. Abraham Maslow, a famous psychologist, described these needs and ranked them in order of importance. Maslow's hierarchy of needs is usually illustrated in a pyramid form with fundamental physiological survival needs having priority over the psychological needs, Figure 2-1.

Maslow believed that people seek to satisfy their physiological needs first. Once these needs are met, people may proceed to fulfill higher-order psychological needs related to emotional and spiritual growth.

Maslow and other psychologists also found that if individuals are confronted with a life-threatening situation, they will defer their psychological needs to only those physiologic needs related to survival. This regression or letting go is linked to the primitive survival instinct. In the face of such events, the needs associated with survival generally take precedence over all other needs.

It is important to remember that a person's sense of belonging and feelings of well-being, security, and self-control may be compromised because of an illness. Showing concern—which can be as simple as being courteous—can help in such situations. Using friendly and encouraging words may help others to cope with stressful circumstances. "How are you feeling today?" "May I help you with your coat and umbrella?" "Please," and "Thank you" are all verbal indicators that you want to help and that you value the other person. A smile helps to show caring and a desire to help others.

All people, and especially patients, seek comfort, reassurance, and answers to their questions. They seek to restore balance to their lives by regaining control. Limited radiographers can meet such patient needs by simply taking time to be understanding.

Suggestions for Relating to Patients

- *Show Concern.* Provide a welcome environment. Show concern by being an empathetic, nonjudgmental person. Concern can be expressed by a touch that shows support and encouragement. Don't hurry the patient or appear rushed to get to the next patient.
- *Show Respect.* Showing respect to others is another way of providing a welcome "We Care" environment. All sexes, races, religions, and socio-economic levels are represented in any patient population. Respect can

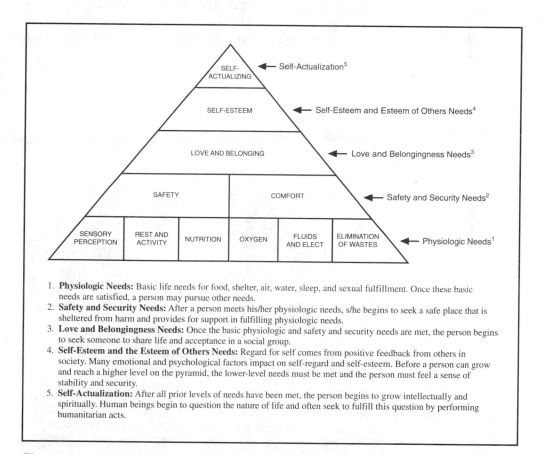

1. **Physiologic Needs:** Basic life needs for food, shelter, air, water, sleep, and sexual fulfillment. Once these basic needs are satisfied, a person may pursue other needs.
2. **Safety and Security Needs:** After a person meets his/her physiologic needs, s/he begins to seek a safe place that is sheltered from harm and provides for support in fulfilling physiologic needs.
3. **Love and Belongingness Needs:** Once the basic physiologic and safety and security needs are met, the person begins to seek someone to share life and acceptance in a social group.
4. **Self-Esteem and the Esteem of Others Needs:** Regard for self comes from positive feedback from others in society. Many emotional and psychological factors impact on self-regard and self-esteem. Before a person can grow and reach a higher level on the pyramid, the lower-level needs must be met and the person must feel a sense of stability and security.
5. **Self-Actualization:** After all prior levels of needs have been met, the person begins to grow intellectually and spiritually. Human beings begin to question the nature of life and often seek to fulfill this question by performing humanitarian acts.

Figure 2-1. Hierarchy of basic needs according to Maslow be verbalized in the way one talks to this diverse population and can be nonverbal via attitude and attention.

■ Treat others as you would want to be treated.
■ Treat all patients equally regardless of their sex, race, religion, or socioeconomic level.
■ Remember children are people too.
■ React professionally to what you see or hear while providing patient care.

Respect and concern can be shown by paying attention to detail — "going the extra mile" or "giving one hundred and ten percent" to perform acts of courtesy. Details, often insignificant in a nonmedical environment, can take on great significance when a person is in a threatening or fearful situation. Loss of identity as an individual, Figure 2-2, and lack of privacy can threaten basic human needs. Use the patient's name and provide personal privacy whenever possible.

Figure 2-2. Professionals' view of patients. Using patients' names instead of calling them by a number, body part, or procedure shows respect and caring for them as individuals. *(From Purtilo, R.* Health Professional/Patient Interactions, *4th ed. Philadelphia: W.B. Saunders Company, 1990, p. 169.)*

A person's needs and perceptions can predict the outcome of relationships and communication. Such needs and perceptions influence whether people are open to positive interpersonal relationships or unconsciously set up barriers. Table 2-1 shows positive and negative styles that have such influences.

Interpersonal Relationships with Coworkers

Limited radiographers work in settings where many other medical personnel are employed. The entire group of employees is called the health care team. This team should work toward the common goal of providing quality professional services and patient care. It is important that all team members work at peak performance levels and do so in an efficient, cooperative manner. However, in any group of employees there is likely to be some disagreement. Disagreement may occur not only because each team member is an individual with very unique personality traits, but also because health care providers perform their daily duties in a work environment that can be very stressful. How, then, can harmony be achieved? To make the team successful every member must make an effort. Important components of this effort are:

TABLE 2–1   ESTABLISHING INTERPERSONAL RELATIONSHIPS

POSITIVE STYLE (Open to Interpersonal Relationships)	NEGATIVE STYLE (Barriers to Interpersonal Relationships)
Silence	Commanding
Open-ended acknowledgment	Threatening
Listening	Advising
Feedback	Lecturing
Assertiveness	Criticizing
Problem-solving approach	Shaming
	Interpreting
	Sympathizing
	Interrogating
	Humoring

- Effective communication
- Respect for one another
- A positive image about each individual's role as it relates to the entire health care team and to the delivery of professional services.

Frequent staff meetings are one way of allowing everyone to communicate and to refocus the group on the team's objectives. Positive relationships with coworkers do not just happen; rather, they result from behaviors and actions that foster a supportive team feeling. The following behaviors and actions can be used to nurture positive coworker relationships:

- Don't become so preoccupied with work that you forget to extend simple courtesies to your coworkers.
- Prepare a birthday list of all employees, and recognize people on their special day. A cake-and-ice-cream break provides an opportunity for the staff to get together in a nonstressful time period.
- If it is office custom to occasionally bring in doughnuts, take your turn and bring them, even if you don't eat them. What matters is an attitude of "I'm one of you" and "We're in this together." Eating healthy? Bring in a low-fat, low-calorie treat.
- Did you take the last cup of coffee in the pot? Make more coffee.
- If you see a coworker overwhelmed with last minute work, such as filing charts or folding statements, pitch in and help.
- Try eating lunch with coworkers instead of alone. Alone is okay, but it sets you off from the group.
- Adopt a "no gossip" attitude. Positive relationships are built on trust; trust cannot survive in a gossip-filled environment.
- Do you have a problem with a particular person? Try talking with that person about how you feel and see if the problem can be resolved.
- Are you unhappy? You don't like or enjoy being with your coworkers? Consider finding a new job.

Interpersonal Relationships with Physicians/Supervisors

A positive work relationship with physicians and immediate supervisors is important. To reach the medical team's objectives, everyone must be able to communicate effectively and be supportive of each other. This cannot occur when there is disrespect or even dislike for one another.

Suggestions:

- Review the suggestions for positive coworker interpersonal relationships; these also apply to physicians and supervisors.

■ Provide positive feedback. Physicians and especially supervisors need to hear that they have done something right or good instead of wrong or bad. If you notice something that physicians or supervisors do that you consider right or good, tell them so. Encouragement and praise can be contagious.

■ Address physicians by their title—"Doctor." This helps maintain a professional atmosphere.

■ Give and expect common courtesy.

■ In conversations with coworkers, patients, or others, reflect an attitude of confidence and support for the physician's professional integrity and ability.

Interpersonal Relationships with Others

Radiographers interact with a variety of people; these include company sales and service representatives, hospital/clinic or medical office staff, service workers, and visitors or patient family members. Everyone should be acknowledged and treated in a pleasant, agreeable manner. Visitors who do not accompany a patient should identify themselves and state the nature of their business. Generally, sales and service representatives or other business people will present a business card and explain the purpose of their visit. Every medical facility will operate differently, so it is necessary to find out how to greet and handle regular business callers and those who are unsolicited.

The key to effective interpersonal relationships with others is to treat each person as a valuable individual and to treat others as you would like to be treated.

Part II:
Communication

INTRODUCTION

In daily life, family members, coworkers, friends, and acquaintances may be able to communicate in loose, imprecise, and familiar ways because the

social-personal history between the communicators is known and the circumstances surrounding the message mutually understood. However, in
medical care settings, communication must be precise and result in understanding and agreement on what is wrong and what must be done as quickly
and accurately as possible. The skill with which communication is accomplished may tilt a delicate relationship or attitude in one crucial direction
or another.

CONCEPTS OF COMMUNICATION

Communication may be defined as the exchange of information between
two persons. The information is called a *message*. The person who communicates first is the *sender*, and the person to whom the communication
is sent is called the *receiver*. The roles of sender and receiver may constantly
change during the course of the interchange. This process is one form of
communication and the receiver is more likely to interpret the information
of the message correctly if the message is simple and precise. The sending
and receiving process can become complicated and information misinterpreted because a person's tone, voice modulation, pauses, and nonverbal
cues can express attitudes and emotions that the words do not convey. For
example, consider the simple message "Close the window." Repeat this
message several times, altering your tone of voice, pauses, and body
language. Note how methods of expression and tone can confuse understanding of the real message. Imagine how a simple message like "Good morning" can be interpreted if the greeter slams a door immediately after the
words are said!

Nonverbal Communication

In this type of communication the message is sent by facial gestures and
body motions. A major issue with nonverbal communication is that these
messages can be misinterpreted by others. One of the most important
nonverbal techniques is eye contact or avoidance of eye contact. In America,
looking the other person "straight in the eye" is considered to be the sign
of an honest, truthful, sincere person. In Japan, eye contact during a conver-
sation, especially between a subordinate and supervisor, would be considered an insult.

Visual messages, such as facial expressions, are a factor in nonverbal
communication and also in self-esteem. For example, facial expressions with
a smile and the eyebrows raised can show happiness and offer reassurance;

likewise, facial expressions with a frown and the head down can express fear and appear evasive or angry.

In addition to considering appropriate facial expressions for the medical environment, it is necessary to think about the radiographer's general verbal attitude. Is it too casual? Is there too much familiarity with patients or team workers? (e.g., "Hi, Honey" or "Turn over, Honey.") This type of familiarity can embarrass patients undergoing radiography procedures. Socializing with coworkers while performing procedures changes the tone of the encounter.

COMMUNICATION FOR THE LIMITED RADIOGRAPHER

Communication, verbal and nonverbal, is how we present ourselves to others. The combination of what you say, how you say it, and your nonverbal cues while you are saying it form the basis of communication and the impression you make on others. The following are examples of everyday work activities that have such impact:

- Introducing yourself to others
- Giving and receiving messages
- Placing and receiving telephone calls
- Using the intercom system
- Consulting with coworkers, physicians, and supervisors
- Consulting with referring physicians and agencies
- Scheduling patients for radiographs
- Responding to patient concerns, questions, and statements
- Giving patients instructions
- Taking patient information
- Explaining radiographic procedures to patients
- Reporting to coworkers, supervisors, and physicians

A radiographer's most important tool is the ability to really observe what is happening when interacting with others. The words *look*, *hear*, and *feel* are very important when dealing with others. One does not have to ask, "How are you?" Observe the other person's complexion, posture, movement, etc.

Introducing Yourself to Others

In the medical environment, you are like a host or hostess. It is part of your job to greet others and introduce yourself. A usual introduction consists of the verbal exchange and nonthreatening body language.

An example of a verbal exchange is "Hello (Good morning, Good afternoon). I am Susan Spencer." Most facilities require that employees wear a name tag that lists name and job title so patients and others can quickly recall the name.

Body language should vary according to the age (or physical condition) of the person to whom you are introducing yourself. Greet adults face to face with an arm's-length distance between yourself and the other person. Distance is important in communication—if you are too close, you may threaten the other person's private space; if you are too far, you may convey a feeling of unfriendliness. Keep your arms and hands down by your side in a relaxed position. Extend your hand if the other person offers to shake hands. When you greet children, get down to the child's height. This technique can also be used for wheelchair patients.

Taking Messages

Health care providers should always have a pen and pad of paper handy so that oral messages can be written down. Commercial message pads are available that list all the essential parts of a message so a critical part will not be omitted—time, date, message content, name, and follow-up directions. Tips for writing messages are:

- Write the message.
- Repeat the message you have just written to check the accuracy of its content.
- Relay or act on the message.

Are you forgetful? If so, keep a bulletin board near your work area. Section off a small area and label messages "To Act On." Check this area several times a day.

Talking with Coworkers, Physicians, and Supervisors

Limited radiographers will talk with coworkers, physicians, and supervisors about many things. It is important to remember that if you have a question about a radiography request or any aspect of a procedure, *never* proceed until you seek assistance. There are situations in which the limited radiographer must seek assistance from the supervisor. Knowing when this is necessary comes from recognizing and understanding the chain of command.

A chain of command, formal or informal, exists in every work environment. The physician is usually the leader and may employ a supervisor to direct and manage the health care team. The physician or supervisor leads the team in providing services and meeting objectives. Limited radiographers may be surrounded by authorities who have varying priorities and time-line expectations. The chain of command concept helps address this confusing situation in a positive way by designating one person as supervisor. The supervisor, who knows the overall goals and objectives, focuses the team's efforts on the priorities to be accomplished. For the chain-of-command concept to work and for all team members to be a functioning part of the group, effective communication and relay of information between and among members must be maintained in a systematic way. A chain of command provides a network system and prevents details and important tasks from being overlooked.

If at any time grievances, complaints, or suggestions need to be discussed, the limited radiographer should take these matters to the immediate supervisor. It is okay to have a grievance or complaint, but the chain of command, not an open public arena, should be used to communicate such issues. Employee, coworker, and supervisor communication, if conducted with candor and a problem-solving attitude (identifying what may be unsatisfactory and correcting it if possible), can be very helpful in improving work relationships. This type of interchange tends to identify and solve problems before they become unsolvable.

Using "I" messages is effective when you are giving criticism, explaining a problem, making a suggestion, or expressing an opinion. "I" messages do not make others feel offended or put them in a defensive position. There are *two* parts to the "I" message: the first part describes your feelings and the second part describes the desired change. The example shown in Table 2-2 illustrates how an "I" message is more effective in communicating a problem than a "You" message.

Talking with Referring Physicians and Agencies

Limited radiographers may have to talk with referring physicians and persons from agencies such as hospitals, nursing homes, or radiology clinics. The following tips should help you perform such tasks efficiently:

- Organize information and questions before contacting the referring physician or agency.

TABLE 2–2 "I" MESSAGES		
"YOU" MESSAGE (Blames Others)	**"I" MESSAGE (First Part) Describes Feelings**	**"I" MESSAGE (Second Part) Describes Desired Change**
"You really make me mad."	"I'm feeling upset about this."	"I would like to talk with you and see if we can't work this out."

- Gather all facts and needed documents.
- Briefly write down key points.
- Make telephone contact.
- Identify yourself, facility, and reasons for the contact.
- Make notes of necessary information. Review with contact.
- Thank contact for his/her time.
- Chart information if necessary.

Responding to Patient Concerns, Questions, and Statements

Limited radiographers are not expected to know all the answers and many times may not be able to release certain information because of confidentiality. However, it is important to always acknowledge patient questions and statements and be perceptive regarding concerns and fears. Effective listening and paraphrasing techniques allow you to respond verbally to patients without appearing curt or that you are withholding the information requested.

Paraphrasing means repeating what a person has said to you but using slightly different words. Paraphrasing a statement helps to determine whether the message has been understood as it was intended, Table 2-3.

Giving Patient Instructions

Limited radiographers often find themselves giving instructions to patients. These instructions may be as simple as where to find the rest room or as complex as how to take self-administered medication for an outpatient

TABLE 2–3 PARAPHRASING	
PATIENT'S STATEMENT	**RADIOGRAPHER'S PARAPHRASE**
"You know, when I fell I hit my knee rather hard and it hurts more than the ankle you are X-raying."	"Are you saying that your knee hurts as much as your ankle?"

examination. The following tips should help you give patients instructions clearly and accurately:

1. Speak slowly.
2. In case of complex instructions, have a written copy of the instructions for the patient. Instructions you give repeatedly to patients should be printed to save time. This also gives patients a handy reference source if they have questions after they leave the facility.
3. Repeat instructions if necessary.
4. Ask the patient to repeat instructions back to you.
5. Ask for questions. Don't appear hurried. Wait. Answer all questions.
6. Never assume that everyone can read.

Taking Patient Information

Patient information is personal and confidential. Provide for privacy. If you must take patient information in an area where others are waiting, be discreet and use a soft voice. Use simple words and double check information. Often, limited radiographers ask questions of a very personal nature, such as (to a female patient), "Could you be pregnant? When was your last menstrual period?" Avoid an unpleasant communication interchange, keep your voice tone low, move closer to the patient to indicate that a question is private. Go further than just the question. You may want to explain briefly how the question relates to radiographic examinations.

Explaining Radiography Procedures to Patients

Limited radiographers need to be able to explain to the patient the nature of the radiography procedures. This usually consists of simple factual information. After identifying the patient as the correct patient, the radiographer may say, "Hello, my name is Elana Brown. I'm going to take the X rays of your right arm that Dr. Christopher ordered." If the patient shows concern over radiation exposure, you will be able to explain briefly how collimation works and give assurance when you place the protective lead apron across the patient's lap.

If at any time the patient indicates an error, such as "It's not my right arm that needs the X ray, it's my left arm," or refuses to have the X-ray examination, STOP and check with your supervisor or the physician. Never proceed with a radiographic procedure if there is a question about the exact nature of the procedure or if the patient refuses.

Mistakes are often made because of miscommunication. Often, this results from not listening to what others are saying. Listening skills are a critical key to effective communication. Limited radiographers need good listening skills not only when receiving directions from physicians and supervisors but also when gathering information and facts from patients and coworkers. Good listeners do not interrupt when others are talking. Also, good listeners use paraphrasing techniques (see Table 2-3) in order to determine if they understand the message.

Reporting to Coworkers, Physicians, and Supervisors

Limited radiographers and other health care providers may be with a patient longer than the physician is and may detect things that need to be reported. If a patient's condition changes during a radiographic procedure, report the change immediately to the physician. Reporting is usually oral but may require written documentation in the patient record. Reporting tips follow.

- Think first. Be specific. What needs to be reported?
- Report to the appropriate person. (*Never* leave a patient unattended while reporting a change in condition.)

RECOGNIZING COMMON BARRIERS TO COMMUNICATION

Ideally, if everyone recognized common barriers to communication, everyday tasks could be achieved with greater understanding and less effort. However, that is not often the case. Limited radiographers especially need to overcome such barriers, not only when barriers originate in the patient, but also when they are self-initiated. A few common barriers to communication are:

- Poor eye contact
- Interrupting the other person before s/he is finished speaking
- Poor listening skills
    Thinking ahead instead of listening
    Pretending to listen
    Misunderstanding
    Ignoring what is said
- Poor oral-verbal skills
    Fear of speaking up
    Rudely disagreeing
    Criticizing instead of explaining

REVIEW QUESTIONS

1. In a written paragraph, discuss the following statement. "Positive interpersonal relationships are established on a foundation of effective communication, both verbal and nonverbal."
2. List and discuss two challenges that limited radiographers may encounter in health care settings that create difficulty in maintaining positive interpersonal relationships and effective communication.
3. Compare and contrast the differences that exist in anxiety or apprehension levels between asymptomatic and symptomatic patients.
4. Briefly discuss the physiological and psychological human needs listed in Abraham Maslow's hierarchy of needs as related to the health care setting.
5. Discuss what is meant by this statement: "A person seeks to satisfy the physiological needs and once these are met may proceed to fulfill the higher-order psychological needs."
6. Discuss one patient care situation in which each of the following positive styles may be used: silence, open-ended acknowledgment, listening, feedback, assertiveness, and problem-solving approach.
7. List several suggestions other than those listed in the chapter that may be used to maintain positive work relationships with coworkers, physicians, supervisors, and others.
8. Discuss how facial expressions and body language can create misinterpretation of the oral communication or send a conflicting message.

BIBLIOGRAPHY

Brewner, Margaret M., William C. McMahon, and Michael P. Roche. *Job Survival Skills*. New York: Educational Designs, Inc., 1984.

Chenevert, Melodie. *Special Techniques in Assertiveness Training for Women in the Health Professions*. St. Louis: C. V. Mosby Co., 1978.

Purtilo, Ruth. *Health Professional/Patient Interactions*. 3d ed. Philadelphia: W. B. Saunders Company, 1984.

CHAPTER

3

Medical Ethics and Law for the Limited Radiographer

CHAPTER OUTLINE

Introduction
Development of a Profession
Definitions of Philosophy and Ethics
  Philosophy
  Ethics
Medical Ethics
  Autonomy
  Beneficence and Nonmaleficence
  Justice
Law for the Radiographer
  Four Types of Law
  Ethical/Legal Behavior
  Codes of Ethics
  Legal/Ethical Definitions
Patients' Rights
Procedural Aspects of Radiology
  Examination Request
  Film Labeling/Identification
  Radiographs as Permanent Records
  Releasing Films
  Informed Consent Forms
  Radiation Safety

OBJECTIVES

Upon completion of the chapter, the student will demonstrate knowledge of the facts and principles presented through oral and written evaluation.

1. Briefly define professional education according to views based on educational philosophy.
2. Identify criteria of a true profession and the relationship of a true profession to ethics and medical ethics.
3. Briefly define philosophy.
4. Define moral ethics, biomedical ethics, and professional ethics.
5. Differentiate between legal/moral concepts.
6. Define given terms applicable to legal radiography issues.
7. Explain the radiographer's code of ethics.
8. Identify and discuss the AMA Patient's Bill of Rights.
9. Describe certain policies and procedures that must be established for performing radiographic procedures.

INTRODUCTION

In his 1960 book *Patterns of Professional Education*, William McGlothlin identified the major focus of professional education in medicine, nursing, law, teaching, social work, and clinical psychology as direct contact with people—people who are patients, students, or clients and who need help solving their problems.[1] He called these professions, very simply, "helping professions." He said that professional education had two aims: (1) to supply enough professional people to help (quantity) and (2) to assure society that they (professionals) are competent (quality).

McGlothlin's philosophy and definition are not obsolete. In 1983 (23 years later), Edmund Pellegrino, in "What is a Profession?" *Journal of Allied Health*, described true professions as those that deal with humans when they are most vulnerable and when they lack the knowledge to make their own decisions. Thus the professional-patient relationship is not of equal power, because generally all the knowledge is on the side of the professional and the need for help is on the patient's side.[2]

Pellegrino further described true professions as being set apart from sociological structures by philosophical definitions. Relatedly, many occupations that were once regarded as crafts, arts, trades, and commerce have developed many elements associated with traditional professions:

■ setting standards for entry
■ defining specific skills or knowledge
■ establishing educational requirements and curriculum

- forming national organizations
- publishing journals
- setting fees and standards for performance
- setting codes of ethics

All of these elements arise from social accountability. The article points out other elements, however, that constitute higher moral and ethical codes. These evolve from philosophical definitions created by the special nature of human relations when people are vulnerable (sick) and in need. It is clear that the fundamental concepts of health professionals and their ethical education change very little in terms of purpose. Before we consider the philosophy that constitutes medical ethics, let us first look at radiography in the professional perspective.

DEVELOPMENT OF A PROFESSION

Professions deal with people and are bound both by sociological structures and by the need to have a higher moral and ethical code that addresses two additional components: (1) ethics and (2) behavior (or manners). Irvin M. Borish states that a true profession evolves in stages and comes to possess three criteria: (1) developed specialized skills, (2) a humane code of ethics, and (3) ethical respect from society as an honorable vocation.[3]

In light of what Borish holds to be criteria for a true profession, does radiography measure up to the definition? With many clinical specialties, administrators, and educators, radiographers form a highly diverse and specialized group. Compared to some other codes of ethics, the code adopted by the radiography profession is very humane and addresses standards of conduct. With regard to respect from society, does society value radiography as an honorable profession? Do people know who radiographers are and what they do? Who communicates that message? Radiographers must communicate the message, each of us, in whatever role we play — general or limited radiographer, specialist, administrator, or educator. No one else will carry the message for us.

DEFINITIONS OF PHILOSOPHY AND ETHICS

Philosophy

Most of us assume that we practice appropriate behavior and that we understand what ethical behavior is. This is generally true in a society that attempts to philosophically understand all behavior and also attempts to teach that understanding. **Philosophy** deals with the search for truth, the general understanding of values and reality. Many areas are included in philosophy: aesthetics (nature of beauty), epistemology (how knowledge is gained), ethics (what is good and bad; moral duty and obligation), and metaphysics (study of what really exists).

Ethics is the area concerned with the examination of human behavior. There are good and bad behavior and there are times when we are bound by a certain duty or obligation. From the time we are old enough to understand, we begin to learn the difference between right and wrong and that we all are expected to use reasonable care in our behavior toward others.

Ethics

By definition, **ethics** refers to the study of human behavior which involves the study of various cultures, religions, groups, and individuals in a systematic way. It is important to try to understand that all persons who require health care will not have the same attitude toward the health care delivery system.

Biomedical ethics, or **bioethics**, involves the knowledge and application of modern medical technologies. **Professional ethics** relates to standards of conduct, dealing with duties, and the rights and obligations of practitioners. It requires that moral judgments and values be based on reason and that individuals carefully consider and take responsibility for their own actions.

MEDICAL ETHICS

If we consider professional codes of ethics as "the rules or standards governing the conduct of the members of a profession"[4] and then think in terms of those members being in the medical profession, we find that many of the rules or standards are general to all disciplines and specialty areas that comprise the medical profession. Although the following discussion does not pretend to address all the rules or standards relevant to ethical behavior for the health care provider, let us look at several elements relevant to medical ethics.

First, a trusting relationship must be established between the patient and the health care provider (radiographer). Some essential elements in building trust are protecting patients' rights at all times, recognizing the psychological state of patients, realizing that each patient is unique, and exhibiting respect and cooperation in interpersonal relationships with patients and other health care providers.

There are four principles on which trusting relationships are based: (1) autonomy, (2) beneficence, (3) nonmaleficence, and (4) justice.

Autonomy

Autonomy is the freedom to govern self and to make one's own decisions according to one's own moral principles. Individual reasons for actions are personal. If we look at each person as an end in himself/herself, then we see that that person has an inherent right to be respected or treated as an autonomous or self-governing individual. In medical ethics, autonomy is viewed as the right of patients to determine what will be done with their own bodies. Two critical elements that arise out of autonomy are informed consent and confidentiality.

Informed Consent.   This is recognized as an individual's right to autonomy. **Informed consent** means that certain standards of disclosure must be followed to assure a patient's full understanding about a medical procedure or treatment. Standards of disclosure include the following, but may vary with facilities:

1. The patient must receive sufficient information in terms s/he can understand.
2. Details of the procedure or treatment must be outlined and discussed.
3. Potential risks and benefits of the procedure or treatment must be disclosed.
4. All available alternatives must be considered and discussed.

Valid informed consent may be determined when:

1. All information according to standards of disclosure has been adequately communicated.
2. The patient has the capacity to understand all information and can make a fair informed decision.
3. Consent for the treatment or procedure is given voluntarily.

Even though the duty of obtaining an informed consent may be delegated to other trained personnel, the physician who is performing the procedure is ultimately responsible for obtaining and assessing that informed consent has been correctly conducted and completed.

Consent of Minors.   Factors that determine whether a minor's consent to a medical or surgical procedure is legally effective are maturity, age of minor, and emancipation. Consent for performing a procedure on a minor must be obtained from a parent or parents or from someone acting in *loco parentis*, i.e., a supervisor or guardian. Emancipation describes a minor who is married or lives independent of a parent or parents (emancipated from his/her parents). Most states do not require parental consent for medical or surgical procedures if the minor is emancipated.

Mental Capacity.   Generally, a person may not be judged competent for reasons of age, mental illness, debilitating disease, or for any other reason that results in diminished capacity to make a rational decision. A person may be declared legally incompetent through a judicial proceeding and a legal guardian appointed where no legal guardian exists and the physician determines the person to be incompetent. Even though the person may give consent, consent from the spouse or nearest relative should also be obtained.

Implied Consent.   Implied consent is an exception to the rule of informed consent. Implied consent refers to a situation in which a person is unconscious or when a life-threatening emergency exists and no one is available to provide legal permission. It may be assumed in such a situation that because it is an emergency, under normal conditions the patient would give consent to save his/her life or to prevent permanent health impairment. If the patient, however, has previously refused treatment prior to the existence of the situation at issue, implied consent is not valid.

Confidentiality.   **Confidentiality** is the patient's basic right to privacy. Confidentiality involves legal as well as ethical considerations. Although not deliberate in many cases, confidentiality is generally the most commonly abused aspect of ethics. Health care providers have a tendency to discuss among themselves what they see and hear. However, they are not expected to discuss any disease or condition or its prognosis with the patient or anyone else. If asked such questions by the patient, the radiographer should explain, "I don't know the answer to that, but your doctor will be happy to discuss it with you."

Beneficence and Nonmaleficence

Beneficence relates to duty to others to provide or improve conditions that promote physical and emotional well-being. **Nonmaleficence** refers to preventing or not causing harm intentionally (i.e., physical assault) or not subjecting another to harm. To illustrate how medical decisions sometimes involve issues of beneficence or nonmaleficence, let us consider the medical professional confronted with the situation of a terminally ill patient. [Can/should enough drugs to reduce the severity of pain to a comfortable stage be given when, if given, the drugs may hasten death or cause drug addiction?] Is it more important that the patient be made comfortable by reducing her/his pain (beneficence) or be put at risk of being harmfully subjected to drug addiction or even early death (nonmaleficence—do no harm)?

Justice

Justice deals with the balancing and fair distribution of medical care, facilities, and resources for society. Simply stated, justice in this sense refers to distributive justice and requires that all economic goods and services be equally distributed unless an unequal distribution would be of greater benefit to all. In some situations, institutions may consider the needs of the poor or those who have less before they consider the needs of more fortunate groups.

LAW FOR THE RADIOGRAPHER

The intent of this chapter is to deal with some legal concepts as they generally apply to health care delivery. To attempt a wide scale, in-depth explanation of the law as it specifically applies to limited radiography in all states would be a major project and beyond the scope of this book. Also, ethical and legal concepts must be situationally applied, according to a particular incident, location, persons involved, and many other elements.

The past several years have seen a steadily increasing need for health care professionals to become knowledgeable about the legal implications of medical practice. In most allied health disciplines, students participating in clinical area learning activities must provide proof of malpractice insurance. Issues relating to malpractice are critical to the health worker. Therefore, it is important to have some general knowledge of the structure of law.

Four Types of Law

There are four types of law: (1) *statutes*, (2) *administrative regulations*, (3) *common law*, and (4) *constitutional law*.

Statutes are laws. They are the principles and rules that are enacted by legislative bodies, such as the Congress of the United States or state legislative bodies. Statutory laws may be amended, expanded, or repealed by the legislative bodies.

Administrative regulations are written by boards or agencies that have been established by legislative bodies for areas where certain kinds of expertise are required to develop specific regulations. Licensing of hospitals, nursing homes, physicians, nurses, and radiographers are some areas where legislators rely on administrative agencies. The regulations are as legally binding as any law the legislators enact.

Common law is a system of applied law and usually develops in the absence of codified written laws or laws enacted through legislation (pertinent statutes). Common law is based on court (i.e., judges') decisions and legal principles and opinion-set precedents considered in those decisions; judges' written opinions often reflect the doctrines of common law. Much common law has evolved over the years and serves to help make decisions in subsequent cases. Common law is legally binding when it is not in conflict with other laws.

Constitutional law is the highest order of law; it is the branch of public law of a nation or state. In matters of constitutional law, the courts do not make law, rather they determine whether a law agrees or is consistent with the constitution of a nation or particular state. If a law is determined to be unconstitutional, it is declared invalid.

Ethical/Legal Behavior

By definition, ethical behavior relates to moral or good conduct, i.e., what is right to do. Legal behavior is what the law or government says we have to do. There are distinctly legal and distinctly moral issues involved in providing medical services. Sometimes what must be done and what should be done become entangled. For example, take the case of a hospital refusing to accept a child who later dies. The hospital had no legal obligation to accept the child, but few people would dispute it may have had a moral obligation to do so. Also consider the case of the physician who has to make the decision to assist or not to assist an injured motorist on the highway. If the physician decides to assist s/he assumes the legal obligation of reasonable care and personal liability. However, even under Good Samaritan laws, which vary from state to state, the physician has no legal obligation to assist. The nature or purpose of a Good Samaritan statute is to encourage voluntary medical assistance to strangers in an emergency situation. Thus, the doctor's decision may depend on ethical or moral values. When health care professionals perform their duties, their actions do have an effect on such issues as patients' autonomy, beneficence, nonmaleficence, and justice;

because these actions involve moral behavior, they sometimes result in problems that require legal answers.

Professional disciplines, such as radiography, are expected to establish their own moral standards of behavior based on common thinking. In light of so much litigation regarding medical procedures, complex modern medical technology, and patients' rights, the trend is that law is becoming more concretely intermingled with codes of ethics.

Codes of Ethics

Two examples of professional codes of ethics are frequently used to illustrate specific standards of professional conduct: the American Medical Association Principles of Medical Ethics and the American Nurses' Association Code. The American Society of Radiologic Technologists Code of Ethics is another specifically written document, Figure 3-1. All three of these documents are good examples of how aspects of duties, ideals, values, and goals of the professional can be expressed. Historically, professional codes have not been utilized and/or may not have contained appropriate language. Such terms as *fairness*, *justice*, *equality*, *duties*, and *rights* have not been used or their meaning has been only vaguely defined. Written codes of ethics are important because they may help bring about professional autonomy, which is appropriate as long as the intent is to better serve and improve the health care delivery system, not to be self-serving.

Currently, there is no code of ethics specifically written for limited radiographers. It would therefore be prudent for limited radiographers to recognize and follow the existing code of ethics written and adopted by the American Society of Radiologic Technologists.

The Code of Ethics for the Profession of Radiologic Technology was developed and adopted by the American Society of Radiologic Technologists and the American Registry of Radiologic Technologists. As you read the Code of Ethics, you should recognize some areas that reflect the previous discussion on the theory of ethics.

Legal/Ethical Definitions

Before briefly discussing the procedural aspects of radiology, some ethical/legal definitions pertinent to limited radiographer interaction with patients and limited radiographer/patient relationships need to be clarified.
Assault. **Assault** is any willful attempt or threat to inflict injury upon the person of another, when coupled with an apparent present ability to do

CODE OF ETHICS*

1. The Radiologic Technologist conducts himself/herself in a professional manner, responds to patient needs and supports colleagues and associates in providing quality patient care.

2. The Radiologic Technologist acts to advance the principal objective of the profession to provide services to humanity with full respect for the dignity of mankind.

3. The Radiologic Technologist delivers patient care and service unrestricted by concerns of personal attributes or the nature of the disease or illness, and without discrimination, regardless of sex, race, creed, religion or socioeconomic status.

4. The Radiologic Technologist practices technology founded upon theoretical knowledge and concepts, utilizes equipment and accessories consistent with the purpose for which they have been designed, and employs procedures and techniques appropriately.

5. The Radiologic Technologist assesses situations, exercises care, discretion and judgement, assumes responsibility for professional decisions, and acts in the best interest of the patient.

6. The Radiologic Technologist acts as an agent through observation and communication to obtain pertinent information for the physician to aid in the diagnosis and treatment management of the patient, and recognizes that interpretation and diagnosis are outside the scope of practice for the profession.

7. The Radiologic Technologist utilizes equipment and accessories, employs techniques and procedures, performs services in accordance with an accepted standard of practice, and demonstrates expertise in limiting the radiation exposure to the patient, self and other members of the health care team.

8. The Radiologic Technologist practices ethical conduct appropriate to the profession, and protects the patient's right to quality radiologic technology care.

9. The Radiologic Technologist respects confidences entrusted in the course of professional practice, protects the patient's right to privacy, and reveals confidential information only as required by law or to protect the welfare of the individual or the community.

10. The Radiologic Technologist continually strives to improve knowledge and skills by participating in educational and professional activities, sharing knowledge with colleagues and investigating new and innovative aspects of professional practice. One means available to improve knowledge and skills is through professional continuing education.

*Reprinted by permission of the American Society of Radiologic Technologists

Figure 3-1. Code of Ethics

so, and any intentional display of force such as would give the victim reason to fear or expect immediate bodily harm.

Battery. **Battery** is any unlawful touching of another which is without justification or excuse.

The ethical concept related to assault and battery is autonomy. Patients must be given full disclosure (informed consent) about what procedure is going to be performed on their bodies. Otherwise, actions toward them could be perceived as intending harm or as touching their bodies without permission.

False Imprisonment. **False imprisonment** is the conscious restraint of the freedom of another without proper authorization, privilege, or consent of that individual.

The ethical concept related to false imprisonment is again autonomy. No one has the right to physically restrain another against his/her will or without permission. The best approach to immobilizing or restraining a patient who may move during exposure is to discuss the procedure directly with the patient. In the case of children, seek parental permission. The two occasions where restraint is justified are (1) when the patient may pose a physical threat to the limited radiographer and (2) when the patient may pose a physical threat to himself/herself.

Negligence. **Negligence** is the omission to do something that a reasonable person (guided by those considerations which ordinarily regulate human affairs) would do, or the doing of something which a reasonable and prudent person would not do.

The related ethical concept deals with the basic duty or obligation to do that which is correct or to behave in a reasonable manner. Negligence is probably the most common cause of litigation. But to prove negligence, the plaintiff must establish four facts: (1) that a duty existed, (2) that a duty was breached, (3) that an injury occurred, and (4) that the breach of duty was the proximate cause of the injury. Negligence is usually determined by assessing how something is customarily done by persons (for example, radiographers) in a similar situation performing a similar procedure (radiographic procedures).

Gross Negligence. **Gross negligence** involves a stronger case of duty. It is intentional failure to perform a manifest duty in reckless disregard of the consequences as affecting the life or property of another.

The related ethical concept is to do no harm, i.e., nonmaleficence. Possibly the strongest determinant for gross negligence is foreseeability. If a situation is clearly a threat or is dangerous to others, and no action is taken to correct the hazard or risk, then one may be held personally accountable for disregard of how others may be affected by a foreseeable hazard.

Defamation.   **Defamation** is the act of bringing harm to another person's reputation through libel (written word) or slander (spoken word).

Defamation is related ethically to confidentiality and is probably the most commonly abused rule of professional conduct. Respecting and protecting the patient's right to privacy (autonomy) is the responsibility of all health care providers. Discussing a patient's medical condition (e.g., AIDS) unnecessarily with another person could be determined as a defamation of character.

Res Ipsa Loquitur.   **Res ipsa loquitur** or "the thing speaks for itself" is a situation where the injured person in no way contributed to her/his injury. That is, the whole incident was under the control of the offender or defendant. Again, negligence becomes obvious.

The ethical concept of nonmaleficence is related to res ipsa loquitur, which is not to cause harm intentionally (negligence) or not to subject another to harm.

PATIENTS' RIGHTS

One of the most important documents to become familiar with in today's health care delivery is the AHA Patient's Bill of Rights, Figure 3-2. The document is based on both the ethical and legal concepts of autonomy and most of its twelve statements deal with confidentiality and informed consent.

PROCEDURAL ASPECTS OF RADIOLOGY

Uppermost in the radiographer's mind is producing not only high-quality diagnostic images but also images of human anatomy that are pleasing to the eye. However, we must take all aspects of the finished radiograph into consideration. Although not limited to this discussion, some of the most important aspects deal with how we produce a radiograph from beginning to end and what could happen during the performance relevant to (1) the examination request, (2) film labeling, (3) film identification, (4) records, (5) retention of records, (6) informed consent forms, (7) radiation safety, (8) equipment safety (refer to compliance regulations and technician certification), and (9) procedure complications. Some of these elements have relevance to our discussion in the earlier part of the chapter, particularly some elements related to autonomy (informed consent and confidentiality), beneficence, and nonmaleficence.

A PATIENT'S BILL OF RIGHTS*

This policy document presents the official position of the American Hospital Association as approved by the Board of Trustees and House of Delegates.

The American Hospital Association presents a Patient's Bill of Rights with the expectation that observance of these rights will contribute to more effective patient care and greater satisfaction for the patient, his physician, and the hospital organization. Further, the Association presents these rights in the expectation that they will be supported by the hospital on behalf of its patients, as an integral part of the healing process. It is recognized that a personal relationship between the physician and the patient is essential for the provision of proper medical care. The traditional physician-patient relationship takes on a new dimension when care is rendered within an organizational structure. Legal precedent has established that the institution itself also has a responsibility to the patient. It is in recognition of these factors that these rights are affirmed.

1. The patient has the right to considerate and respectful care.
2. The patient has the right to obtain from his physician complete current information concerning his diagnosis, treatment, and prognosis in terms the patient can be reasonably expected to understand. When it is not medically advisable to give such information to the patient, the information should be made available to an appropriate person in his behalf. He has the right to know, by name, the physician responsible for coordinating his care.
3. The patient has the right to receive from his physician information necessary to give informed consent prior to the start of any procedure and/or treatment. Except in emergencies, such information for informed consent should include but not necessarily be limited to the specific procedure and/or treatment, the medically significant risks involved, and the probable duration of incapacitation. Where medically significant alternatives for care or treatment exist, or when the patient requests information concerning medical alternatives, the patient has the right to such information. The patient also has the right to know the name of the person responsible for the procedures and/or treatment.
4. The patient has the right to refuse treatment to the extent permitted by law and to be informed of the medical consequences of his action.
5. The patient has the right to every consideration of his privacy concerning his own medical care program. Case discussion, consultation, examination, and treatment are confidential and should be conducted discreetly. Those not directly involved in his care must have the permission of the patient to be present.
6. The patient has the right to expect that all communications and records pertaining to his care should be treated as confidential.
7. The patient has the right to expect that within its capacity a hospital must make reasonable response to the request of a patient for services. The hospital must provide evaluation, service, and/or referral as indicated by the urgency of the case. When medically permissible, a patient may be transferred to another facility only after he has received complete information and explanation concerning the needs for and alternatives to such a transfer. The institution to which the patient is to be transferred must first have accepted the patient for transfer.
8. The patient has the right to obtain information as to any relationship of his hospital to other health care and educational institutions insofar as his care is concerned. The patient has the right to obtain information as to the existence of any professional relationships among individuals, by name, who are treating him.
9. The patient has the right to be advised if the hospital proposes to engage in or perform human experimentation affecting his care or treatment. The patient has the right to refuse to participate in such research projects.
10. The patient has the right to expect reasonable continuity of care. He has the right to know in advance what appointment times and physicians are available and where. The patient has the right to expect that the hospital will provide a mechanism whereby he is informed by his physician or a delegate of the physician of the patient's continuing health care requirements following discharge.
11. The patient has the right to examine and receive an explanation of his bill regardless of source of payment.
12. The patient has the right to know what hospital rules and regulations apply to his conduct as a patient.

No catalog of rights can guarantee for the patient the kind of treatment he has a right to expect. A hospital has many functions to perform, including the prevention and treatment of disease, the education of both health professionals and patients, and the conduct of clinical research. All these activities must be conducted with an overriding concern for the patient, and, above all, the recognition of his dignity as a human being. Success in achieving this recognition assures success in the defense of the rights of the patient.

---

*From Hegner & Caldwell. NURSING ASSISTANT: A NURSING PROCESS APPROACH, 6th Edition, Delmar Publishers. 1992. ISBN 4800-2. Figure 3-1, page 28.

Figure 3-2. A Patient's Bill of Rights

Examination Request

Before ever seeing the patient, the radiographer receives an examination request that has been written by the patient's attending physician. Items included on the requisition include the patient's name and vital statistics, the type of radiographic procedure to be performed (e.g., chest), why it needs to be done (history), and the doctor's signature.

A common practice is for the radiographer to ask the female patient who is of appropriate (childbearing) age when she had her last menstrual period (LMP). The information should be written on the request; some practitioners prefer to have the patient's personal signature in the LMP area of request. Where this is the policy and a patient is unable to sign her name, the attending physician or a guardian may sign for her.

The limited radiographer is clearly placed in a decision-making position when reading the examination request (1) to make sure signatures are appropriate, (2) to assure that critical questions have been asked, and (3) to determine that the patient's medical history relating to the radiographic examination is written on the request. The information included on an examination request is critical to making sure that the proper examination is done and that the radiologist has sufficient background information to aid in interpreting the radiographic image. Although examination requests are more commonly computer-generated in most radiology office and hospital departments, an example is included in Figure 3-3.

Film Labeling/Identification

Film labeling, using lead letters to indicate the patient's identification and that the correct side of the body has been marked, is crucial. If a film has no markings on it, it really belongs to no one and therefore has no value and should be discarded. If for some reason, a film was not labeled at the time it was taken, it must be marked immediately after processing. Legally, the markings should be put on the film in a permanent manner (e.g., a black felt pen). This shows there was no intent of deception and that the one who marked the film can demonstrate that the markings are clearly correct.

Radiographs as Permanent Records

Radiographs are permanent records. Although the information contained in records is subject to the patient's use, the records belong to the office or institution where they were made. It is therefore important that these records be accurately maintained for future purposes. Some important reasons are:

APPT. #	CURR. X-RAY #	NAME		TODAY'S DATE	TIME	PAGE

BIRTH DATE	AGE	M/F	HOSPITAL #	EMER. REC. #	

ADDRESS 1		ADDRESS 2	CITY	STATE	ZIP

HOME PHONE	WORK PHONE	HOSP. ROOM	BED	SCHED. BY	CHANGED BY

REFERRING PHYSICIAN 1	REFERRING PHYSICIAN 2

RADIOLOGIST	10E	TRANSPORT	ADMITTING DIAGNOSIS

APPOINTMENT REMARKS	PREGNANT	LMP	DEPARTMENT	

SPECIAL HANDLING

TECH	# FILMS	FILM TYPE	TECH NOTES

PAT RQST	PAT ARVL	EXAM START	EXAM END	LEFT DEPT	

PREVIOUS EXAMS

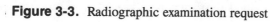

Figure 3-3. Radiographic examination request

(1) follow-up for certain diseases or conditions, e.g., cancer, emphysema; (2) annual physical, e.g., chest examinations; (3) legal procedures, such as in trauma cases; and (4) research and teaching. Appropriate policies and procedures must be established for not losing films when they are loaned to doctors or other persons (i.e., lawyers). There also must be policies established regarding films subpoenaed for litigation. These kinds of policies are a protection for everyone involved. (See sample release form, Figure 3-4.)

Releasing Films

The following procedures are suggested for releasing films from the office or department to other physicians, the patient, or other than medical personnel.

1. *Other physicians*—a release form must be filled out by the patient. The films may be transferred to a different film jacket to be sent out. (Until the films are returned, the original film jacket and reports are refiled.) The jacket for sending out should be stamped *Please Return to* with your office name and address provided (like a self-addressed reply envelope).
2. *The patient*—the patient must fill out a release form and sign it. The doctor to whom the patient is taking the film should be notified. When the films have served the intended purpose, they must be returned to the proper office or department.
3. *Other than medical personnel*—this category includes such persons as lawyers and insurance company personnel. A release/consent form must be filled out by the patient and/or the physician.

The best method for record keeping today is through computerized programs so that standard procedures and accuracy may be ensured. The length of time that medical records must be kept depends on state regulations regarding medical records. Generally five years of current films are kept in files and then purged for storage or discard. If films are of minors, the length of time they must be kept may be longer than five years. Radiology records also provide information for administrative reports. A daily log of appointments and procedures is generally maintained; billing is indicated for examinations completed. Quality control reports are generated to show film usage and numbers and types of procedures completed.

Informed Consent Forms

Informed consent forms must always be available and limited radiographers must be educated in their appropriate use. Informed consents should

REQUEST FOR RELEASE OF RADIOGRAPHIC FILM

Request is made by the undersigned patient to review personal radiographic films on file at
_____ Hospital/Clinic.

_____
DATE

_____
SIGNATURE OF PATIENT

PATIENT'S SS# _____

_____
SIGNATURE OF PERSON AUTHORIZING RELEASE

Film Record Room Information:

_____
PATIENT'S NAME (PRINTED)

_____
SIGNATURE OF RADIOLOGIST

FILM REPORT INCLUDED: YES _____   NO _____

PURPOSE OF RELEASE _____

_____

_____
DATE REMOVED

_____
PERSON RELEASING

_____
DATE RETURNED

Figure 3-4. Sample release form

PATIENT'S CONSENT STATEMENT FOR RADIOGRAPHIC PROCEDURE

I, _____ , understand that my doctor, _____
(physician performing procedure)

has ordered a _____ which requires the injection or introduction of
(type of procedure)

_____ into my body for diagnostic purposes.
(contrast medium)

I have answered the following questions as far as I know them to be true according to my personal knowledge.

Are you allergic to any types of: medication ☐   food ☐   shellfish ☐   other ☐

If so, what? _____

_____

Have you ever had any of the following? (Check all that apply)

☐ Asthma   ☐ Diabetes   ☐ Neurological Problems
☐ Cardiac (Heart) Disease   ☐ Renal (Kidney) Disease   ☐ Do not know

If you have had this radiographic procedure before or any similar type procedure that included an injection, did you have any problems after the injection?

_____

_____

After reading and discussing this form, and having my questions answered satisfactorily by the physician performing the procedure, I voluntarily consent to the injection of contrast medium for the following procedure: _____

_____   Date: _____
(Signature of Patient)

Witness: _____

Patient is unable to consent because: _____

_____

_____   Date: _____
(Signature of legal guardian or
closest available relative)

Witness: _____   Witness: _____

Note. This is a sample only. Consent forms are designed for specific use and must be checked with legal counsel before use. Consent forms should be obtained by the performing physician or other qualified persons trained in managing such procedures.

Figure 3-5. Sample informed consent form

be written so that persons from all levels of education may understand them. The forms should indicate that the patient has been appropriately informed about the risks, benefits, and alternatives with regard to the procedure to be performed on the patient's body. If the duty has been delegated by the physician, the limited radiographer should make sure the consent form has been signed and is in the patient's record for review by the physician prior to doing the radiographic procedure. If the form is not appropriately completed, medical personnel and the office or institution involved in performing the procedure may be subject to legal action should any mistakes or unexpected events occur. (See sample consent form, Figure 3-5.)

Radiation Safety

Radiation safety must be in compliance with (1) the National Council on Radiation Protection and Measurements (NCRP), which is a regulatory agency for evaluating the relationship between radiation exposure and biological effects; and (2) the Consumer-Patient Radiation Health and Safety Act of 1981 (refer to chapter 1), which deals with the establishment of minimum standards for accreditation of radiologic technology programs for persons who administer radiographic procedures. Radiation safety procedures must be written and documentation of equipment inspections must be kept on file at the office or facility.

REVIEW QUESTIONS

1. Ethics is concerned with
   a) nature of beauty
   b) what really exists
   c) human behavior
   d) knowledge gained
2. Professional ethics relates to
   a) modern technology
   b) standards of conduct
   c) metaphysics
   d) truth
3. The freedom to govern self is based on
   a) justice
   b) autonomy
   c) confidentiality
   d) beneficence

4. The person legally responsible for obtaining and assessing correct informed consent is the
   a) limited radiographer
   b) patient
   c) physician performing the procedure
   d) referring physician
5. The patient's basic right to privacy is based on
   a) type of illness
   b) informed decision
   c) confidentiality
   d) beneficence
6. Nonmaleficence refers to
   a) disclosing information
   b) doing duty toward others
   c) distributing fairly
   d) doing no harm
7. Principles and rules enacted by legislative bodies are
   a) common law
   b) statutes
   c) administrative regulations
   d) none of the above
8. Fairness, justice, duties, rights, and equality are terms that should be used to develop
   a) administrative regulations
   b) disclosure of information
   c) codes of ethics
   d) all of the above
9. Unlawful touching of another without permission is
   a) battery
   b) assault
   c) negligence
   d) false imprisonment
10. Conscious restraint of freedom is
    a) negligence
    b) defamation
    c) false imprisonment
    d) battery

REFERENCES ▬▬▬▬▬▬▬▬▬▬▬▬▬▬▬▬▬▬▬▬▬▬▬▬▬▬▬▬

1. McGlothlin, William. *Patterns of Professional Education*. New York: Putnam, 1960.
2. Pellegrino, Edmund. "What Is A Profession?" *Journal of Allied Health* 12, no. 3 (1983).
3. Borish, Irvin M. "The Academy and Professionalism," *The American Journal of Optometry & Physiological Optics*, 1983.
4. *The American Heritage Dictionary* (2d College Edition). Boston: Houghton Mifflin Company, 1982, p. 467.

BIBLIOGRAPHY ▬▬▬▬▬▬▬▬▬▬▬▬▬▬▬▬▬▬▬▬▬▬▬▬▬▬▬

Anderson, Gray R. and Valerie A. Anderson-Glesnes. *Health Care Ethics*. Rockville, MD: Aspen Publishers, Inc., 1987.

Arras, John and Nancy Rhoden. *Ethical Issues in Modern Medicine*. 3d ed. Mountain View, CA: Mayfield Publishing Company, 1989.

Bayles, Michael D. *Professional Ethics* 2d ed. Belmont, CA: Wadsworth Publishing Co., 1989.

Beauchamp, Tom L. and LeRoy Walters. *Contemporary Issues in Bioethics* 3d ed. Belmont, CA: Wadsworth Publishing Company, 1989.

Pozgar, George D. *Legal Aspects of Health Care Administration*. Rockville, MD: Aspen Publications, 1987.

CHAPTER

4

Medical Asepsis and Patient Care

CHAPTER OUTLINE

The Patient's Record: A Resource Document
  Making Entries on Patient Records
Meeting Patient's Needs
  Physical Needs
  Other Needs
IV Tubes, Urinary Catheters, Nasal Oxygen
Vital Signs
  Temperature
  Pulse
  Respiration
  Blood Pressure
Medical Emergencies
  Fainting
  Seizures
  Nosebleeds

OBJECTIVES

Upon completion of the chapter, the student will meet the following objectives by verifying knowledge of the facts and principles presented through oral and written communication at a level deemed competent and meet the task objectives by demonstrating the specific behavior as identified in the terminal performance objectives of the procedures.

1. Describe the limited radiographer's role in preventing the spread of microorganisms.
2. Recall and outline the requirements for microbial growth.
3. Differentiate between the levels of infection control by comparing and contrasting methods and uses of medical asepsis, disinfection, and surgical asepsis.
4. Recall the Centers for Disease Control's recommendations for prevention of HIV, hepatitis B, and other communicable diseases.
5. Identify common safety measures that the limited radiographer can practice.
6. Identify principles of body mechanics and relate these to radiographer and patient safety and comfort.
7. Identify the common vital signs and describe their importance in the assessment of patient conditions.
8. Identify normal vital sign ranges for adults and children, to include temperature, pulse, respiration, and blood pressure.

9. Discriminate between appropriate and inappropriate procedures and techniques related to taking and recording vital signs, administering oxygen, responding to emergencies, and handling trauma patients.
10. Define what constitutes a medical emergency and identify the limited radiographer's role.
11. Demonstrate competence in each task listed below. Refer to the appendix for the individual procedure/performance guides.

TASKS (See Appendix):

4-1 Hand Washing
4-2 Assisting the Falling Patient
4-3 Preparing Safety Reports (Accident/Incident)
4-4 Transferring the Patient Using a Three-Carrier Lift
4-5 Transferring a Patient Using a Sheet
4-6 Logrolling the Patient
4-7 Assisting the Patient with Ambulatory Aid: Cane, Walker, and Crutches
4-8 Transporting the Patient in a Wheelchair
4-9 Transferring the Patient between Radiographic Table and Wheelchair
4-10 Preparing Patient for Radiographic Examination
4-11 Taking Temperature by Mercury and Electronic Thermometers
4-12 Counting the Radial Pulse and Respiratory Rate
4-13 Taking Blood Pressure

INTRODUCTION

Today, health care is provided in a variety of settings, from hospitals offering a wide range of services to those providing specialized care, such as community health agencies, private medical offices, mobile van care units, ambulatory emergency clinics, nursing homes, hospices, and self-help organizations. Home health care is becoming a vital service in the health care industry; so are health maintenance organizations, which stress a holistic wellness approach. Rehabilitation is also very important today to help people return to an active life after an accident or illness.

The traditional objectives of medical science—prevention, detection, and treatment of disease—remain the foundations for delivery of health care. However, ethical, moral, and legal debates are taking issue with procedures used to initiate, prolong, and redesign the life process. As scientific advances continue to expand the role and scope of health care, these and other ethical and legal questions concerning rights and responsibilities will continue to be addressed.

Despite these unanswered questions and the turmoil they bring to the entire health care community, the everyday needs of patients seeking health care must be served. The limited radiographer's primary responsibility is to provide diagnostic-quality radiographs as requested by a licensed practitioner of the healing arts. Because of the nature of the work, limited radiographers also give basic patient care and have an important role in the entire process of health care delivery.

INFECTION CONTROL

Medical institutions, clinics, doctors' offices, and others provide services to many people. **Infection control**, i.e., the prevention of the spread of infectious conditions and diseases, is an important responsibility and goal for everyone. Consider the unlimited possibilities for disease transmission and cross infection between and among the many people who enter a medical facility. Infection can spread from a single focal point or person of contamination to many other parts of the medical care chain and the general public, Figure 4-1.

Limited radiographers are responsible for preventing the spread of microorganisms to others and for protecting themselves from contamination. By consistent application of basic techniques of hand washing, proper disinfection, and disposal of contaminated items, the total number of infectious organisms can be reduced or diluted to a harmless level.

The goal then becomes to protect self, patient, and others from becoming infected and from serving as a source of infectious organisms to others.

MICROORGANISMS

The environment is teeming with **microorganisms,** which are extremely small and invisible except by microscope. Microorganisms also reside on all skin surfaces of the body and are especially numerous in the respiratory passages, mouth, and entire length of the digestive system. Not all microorganisms are harmful; microorganisms that are not harmful are called **nonpathogenic.** Those that are harmful and capable of causing diseases are referred to as **germs** or **pathogenic organisms**. The five general classifications of microorganisms are *bacteria, fungi, protozoa, rickettsiae,* and *viruses.*

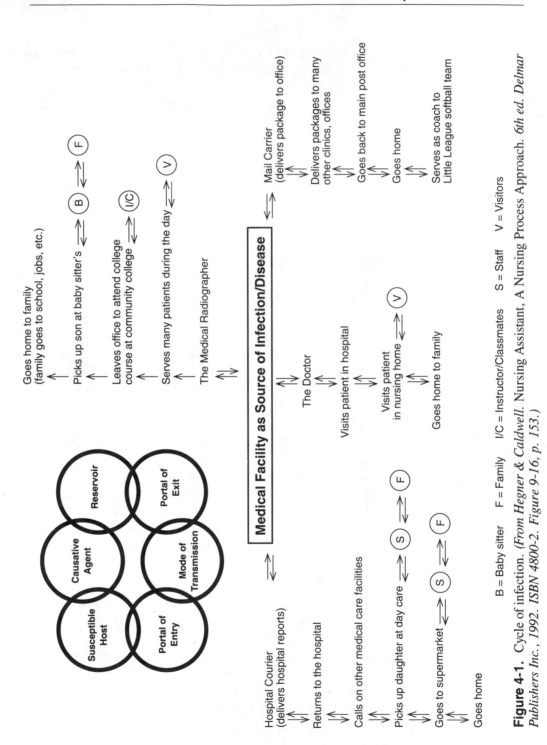

Figure 4-1. Cycle of infection. *(From Hegner & Caldwell. Nursing Assistant, A Nursing Process Approach. 6th ed. Delmar Publishers Inc., 1992. ISBN 4800-2. Figure 9-16, p. 153.)*

Bacteria

Bacteria are one-celled organisms, both pathogenic and nonpathogenic, and are identified and classified according to their morphology (shape) and structure.

Fungi

Fungi exist in two forms, yeasts and molds. Yeasts are one-celled animals, whereas molds are multicelled. Approximately fifty percent of all fungi may cause disease in humans. Fungi require moisture and darkness to survive and are often called opportunistic because they are not particularly pathogenic until they encounter a compromised host. Fungi infections occur under numerous conditions and may be a symptom of a more serious disease or infection. Common fungal diseases are thrush, moniliasis, and histoplasmosis.

Protozoa

Protozoa are microscopic one-celled animals. Infection occurs as a result of ingestion of the parasite or from an insect/animal bite. Examples of protozoal diseases are amebiasis, malaria, and toxoplasmosis.

Rickettsiae

Rickettsiae are microscopic life forms found in tissues of fleas, lice, ticks, and other insects. Rickettsial infections are transmitted to humans by the bite of infected insects, which are called a **vector** or the carrier of disease. Common examples of rickettsial diseases are typhus and Rocky Mountain spotted fever.

Viruses

Viruses are the smallest known organisms. Viruses cannot exist outside a living cell and can only be seen by means of the electron microscope. Humans are susceptible to several hundred different viruses. Common virus infections are influenza, measles, German measles, mumps, chicken pox, herpes simplex, and smallpox. Because of their prevalence, viruses are an important consideration in infection control. They are spread primarily by humans via respiratory and intestinal excretions.

NOSOCOMIAL INFECTIONS

Nosocomial infections are often called opportunistic infections. The term is used to describe a group of infections caused by resistant and extremely pathogenic bacteria. These infections occur in hospitals and medical care settings and cause wound, urinary, and upper respiratory infections. They are considered opportunistic since they are more likely to occur in persons with weakened immune defenses due to injury, disease, or long-term antibiotic or corticosteroid drug use. Common opportunistic infections are caused by *Staphylococcus* bacteria ("Staph"), *Escherichia coli*, and *pseudomonas aeruginosa*. Nosocomial infections are spread more by hands than any other method, so proper hand washing can reduce their spread.

MICROBIAL GROWTH AND INFECTION

Microorganisms have certain specific requirements for growth. Knowing these requirements will help the radiographer recognize and eliminate conditions conducive to microbial growth. In this way, the spread of infection to others can be inhibited.

REQUIREMENTS FOR GROWTH:

1. **Host** or reservoir in which to live and grow. The host can be a human being, animal, soil, water, or food. Hosts must provide water and nourishment for the microorganisms.
2. Warm and dark environment. Most microorganisms grow best at body temperature (98.6 degrees Fahrenheit) and prefer a dark environment.

Microorganisms can be spread by a number of methods, Figure 4-2. Infection is caused when microorganisms enter a susceptible host and grow in the body. An infection can be localized or affect the entire body. The factors involved in the process of infection are:

- source of infection (reservoir)
- the microorganisms (causative agent)
- a portal of exit from the reservoir
- a host with a level of susceptibility and a portal of entry

Direct spread of microorganisms occurs when the microorganisms are passed from one person to another by touching or contact. Indirect spread of microorganisms involves the transmission of pathogens by one of three means:

1. Fomites: A **fomite** is an object that has been contaminated with the pathogen. Common examples are a limited radiographer's uniform or the radiographic table. Common fomites are doors, examination tables, equipment, and hypodermic needles.

2. Vector: A **vector** is an animal or insect whose body serves as host to the pathogen. The bite of the infected vector spreads the disease.

Disease	Vector
Rabies	Bats, dogs, etc.
Bubonic Plague	Fleas
Rat bite fevers	Rats
Malaria	Mosquitoes

3. Airborne: **Airborne pathogens** are spread by dust or droplet contamination. This occurs when infected individuals sneeze or cough toward a susceptible host.

Figure 4-2. Methods of spreading microorganisms

Remember the following important facts about microorganisms as they relate to the spread of infection:

- Microorganisms are everywhere in our environment.
- Microorganisms cannot move by themselves, but must be transported from one host to another.
- Microorganisms are opportunistic.
- Severity of infection depends on:
    number of pathogenic organisms present
    virulence (strength) of organisms
    resistance of infected person

The human body's defenses are usually strong enough to protect against invading opportunistic microorganisms. However, those seeking health care may have a medical condition or a compromised immune system that leaves them with reduced defenses against the attack.

LEVELS OF INFECTION CONTROL

Infection control includes various actions and procedures that reduce or eliminate the number of pathogenic organisms present. There are three levels of infection control: asepsis, disinfection, and surgical asepsis.

Asepsis

Asepsis is defined as the absence of all disease-producing microorganisms and is very important to breaking the infection cycle. Aseptic techniques physically eliminate pathogens and the conditions that promote their growth and spread. Such techniques include proper hand washing, handling and disposing of contaminated linens, and housekeeping.

Hand Washing. The hands are a limited radiographer's tools. Radiographers constantly use their hands to prepare the examination room and equipment, to assist and position the patient, and to perform all the tasks associated with providing radiographs. During these tasks, the hands are exposed to pathogens that can infect the limited radiographer, who, in turn, can become a reservoir of infection passed on to others. For this reason, individuals providing medical care should not wear rings (except for a simple wedding band) or have chipped nail polish because these may be contaminated by pathogenic microorganisms.

To prevent the spread of infectious microorganisms hands must be washed frequently, such as before and after working with each patient. It may be necessary to wash hands several times during the period of patient contact for a specific radiographic procedure. In addition to frequent hand washing, any cut or break in the skin should be covered with a sterile dressing. Since dry, chapped, or abraded skin also serves as a portal of entry for micro-organisms, care should be taken to keep the skin smooth and intact. **Refer to Task 4-1 in the appendix for the hand washing procedure.**

Handling and Disposing of Linens.   All used linen should be considered soiled and a source of pathogenic microorganisms. The use of disposable gowns, sheets, drapes, and pillow covers eliminates risks associated with cleaning and reuse of linens. Used linen, whether disposable or non-disposable, should be handled as little as possible and with minimum movement to prevent contamination of the air and of persons handling the linen, Figure 4-3.

Figure 4-3. Handling linens. Linens should be unfolded, never flipped or fanned, because brisk movement stirs up air currents that carry microorganisms into the air.

All used linen should be bagged at the location where it is used. Do not sort or rinse linens in the patient care area. Linens soiled with blood or body fluids should be placed and transported in bags that prevent leakage.

Housekeeping. Housekeeping activities include cleaning environmental surfaces such as walls, floors, and other surfaces. Because these surfaces are not directly associated with the transmission of microorganisms to patients or others, attempts to disinfect or sterilize are not necessary; however, regular cleaning and soil removal must be performed.

Cleaning schedules and methods vary according to the type of medical facility, the particular service area, and the amount and type of soil present. Furniture and hard surfaced floors should be cleaned on a regular basis and when soiling or spills occur. Walls, window coverings, and blinds should be cleaned when they are visibly soiled. Vigorous cleaning and scrubbing with a disinfectant-detergent formula is considered effective against growth of microorganisms.

Disinfection

Disinfection is the destruction of microorganisms by using chemical methods. In radiography, disinfection methods are used on the radiographic table and certain equipment, accessories, and noninvasive articles. Commercially available disinfectant solutions may be used, but a solution of sodium hypochlorite (household bleach) is an inexpensive and effective germicide. Concentrations ranging from 1:100 dilution of household bleach to water are effective depending on the amount of organic material present on the surface. Regardless of the type or brand of disinfectant solution used, the following recommendations apply. (Information on specific label claims of commercial germicides can be obtained by writing to the Disinfectants Branch, Office of Pesticides, EPA, 401 M Street SW, Washington, DC 20460).

1. Read the directions provided for preparing and using disinfectants.
2. In patient-care areas, visible material should first be removed and then the area should be decontaminated. With large spills of cultured or concentrated infectious agents, the contaminated area should be flooded with a liquid germicide before cleaning, then decontaminated with a fresh germicidal chemical. Gloves should be worn during all cleaning and decontaminating procedures.

Common radiography items that require disinfection are the radiography table top as well as calipers, cassette surfaces, and immobilization aids.

Surgical Asepsis

Surgical asepsis includes procedures and techniques used to destroy microorganisms before they enter the body. Such aseptic techniques are used whenever a surgical incision is made in the body. They are also used with invasive procedures, such as urinary catheterization, and when sterile instruments are handled and dressings are changed.

Surgical asepsis means that everything coming in contact with the patient is sterile. If an article is touched by an unsterile item, or if there is any question about the sterility of an item, it must be considered contaminated. Surgical asepsis is not generally used in procedures related to limited radiography procedures. For further information on surgical asepsis procedures, consult available nursing, health, and health assistant textbooks, which generally include donning sterile gloves, gowning, and preparing a sterile field.

RECOMMENDATIONS FOR THE PREVENTION OF THE SPREAD OF HUMAN IMMUNODEFICIENCY VIRUS (HIV)

AIDS and hepatitis B are just two of the many diseases that health care providers encounter in their daily work. The following suggestions include effective infection control measures for most other pathogens as well as HIV and hepatitis B. The suggestions are taken from the "Recommendations for Prevention of HIV Transmission in Health-Care Settings," published in the U.S. Department of Health and Human Services Centers for Disease Control publication, *Morbidity and Mortality Weekly Report*,[1] and "Update: Universal Precautions for Prevention of Transmission of Human Immunodeficiency Virus, Hepatitis B Virus, and Other Bloodborne Pathogens in Health-Care Settings."[2]

"Human immunodeficiency virus (HIV), the virus that causes acquired immunodeficiency syndrome (AIDS), is transmitted through sexual contact and exposure to infected blood or blood components and perinatally from mother to neonate. HIV has been isolated from blood, semen, vaginal secretions, saliva, tears, breast milk, cerebrospinal fluid, amniotic fluid, and urine and is likely to be isolated from other body fluids, secretions, and excretions. However, epidemiologic evidence has implicated only blood, semen, vaginal secretions, and possibly breast milk in transmission.

"The increasing prevalence of HIV increases the risk that health-care workers will be exposed to blood from patients infected with HIV, especially when blood and body-fluid precautions are not followed for all patients. *Thus health-care workers should consider all patients as potentially infected with HIV and/or other blood-borne pathogens and to adhere rigorously to infection-control precautions for minimizing the risk of exposure to blood and body fluids of all patients.*

"Universal Blood and Body Fluid Precautions

1. All health-care workers should routinely use appropriate barrier precautions to prevent skin and mucus-membrane exposure when contact with blood or other body fluids of any patient is anticipated. Gloves should be worn for touching blood and body fluids, mucus membranes, or non-intact skin of all patients, for handling items or surfaces soiled with blood or body fluids, and for performing venipuncture. Gloves should be changed after contact with each patient. Masks and protective eyewear or face shields should be worn during procedures that are likely to generate droplets of blood or other body fluids to prevent exposure of mucous membranes of the mouth, nose, and eyes. Gowns or aprons should be worn during procedures that are likely to generate splashes of blood or other body fluids.

2. Hands and other skin surfaces should be washed immediately and thoroughly if contaminated with blood or other body fluids. Hands should be washed immediately after gloves are removed.

3. All health-care workers should take precautions to prevent injuries caused by needles, scalpels, and other sharp instruments or devices during procedures; when cleaning used instruments; during disposal of used needles; and when handling sharp instruments after procedures. To prevent needle-stick injuries, needles should not be recapped, purposely bent or broken by hand, removed from disposable syringes, or otherwise manipulated by hand. After they are used, disposable syringes and needles, scalpel blades, and other sharp items should be placed in puncture-resistant containers for disposal; the puncture-resistant containers should be located as close to the use area as practical. Large-bore reusable needles should be placed in a puncture-resistant container for transport to the reprocessing area.

4. Although saliva has not been implicated in HIV transmission, to minimize the need for emergency mouth-to-mouth resuscitation, mouthpieces, masks, resuscitation bags, or other ventilation devices should be available for use in areas in which the need for resuscitation is predictable.

5. Health-care workers who have exudative lesions or weeping dermatitis

should refrain from all direct patient care and from handling patient-care equipment until the condition resolves.

6. Pregnant health-care workers are not known to be at greater risk of contracting HIV infection than health-care workers who are not pregnant; however, if a health-care worker develops HIV infection during pregnancy, the infant is at risk of infection resulting from perinatal transmission. Because of this risk, pregnant health-care workers should be especially familiar with and strictly adhere to precautions to minimize the risk of HIV transmission."

Implementation of universal blood and body-fluid precautions for *all* patients eliminates the need for use of the isolation category of "Blood and Body Fluid Precautions" previously recommended by the Centers for Disease Control (CDC) for patients known or suspected to be infected with blood-borne pathogens.

Implementation of Recommended Precautions

Employers of health-care workers should ensure that policies exist for:

1. Initial orientation and continuing education and training of all health-care workers—including students and trainees—on the epidemiology, modes of transmission, and prevention of HIV and other blood-borne infections and the need for routine use of universal blood and body-fluid precautions for *all* patients.
2. Provision of equipment and supplies necessary to minimize the risk of infection with HIV and other blood-borne pathogens (gloves, gowns, masks, etc.).
3. Monitoring adherence to recommended protective measures. When monitoring reveals a failure to follow recommended precautions, counseling, education, and/or retraining should be provided, and, if necessary, appropriate disciplinary action should be considered.

Professional associations and labor organizations, through continuing education efforts, should emphasize the need for health-care workers to follow recommended precautions.

SAFETY MEASURES

Safety is the responsibility of everyone and must be an integral part of health care services. This concern includes not only the patient, but extends to everyone entering the health care facility. Accidents involving patients and staff can be reduced if simple safety measures are followed.

Preventing Falls

Patients may misjudge the distance from the radiographic examination table to the floor and fall as they attempt to get on and/or off the table. To reduce the likelihood of patient falls, you should always be at the table and provide a foot stool. Provide assistance also when the patient is getting on and off the table.

Tripping and falling account for numerous accidents. Protruding objects, loose scatter rugs, electrical cords, etc., should be removed or secured to prevent injuries. **Refer to Task 4-2 in the appendix, Assisting the Falling Patient.**

Fire Safety

Fire safety begins with a fire safety plan that includes learning the location of fire doors, escape routes, and fire extinguishers, and knowing the evacuation procedure to follow during drills or the real thing. For further information, ask your supervisor about the facility's fire safety plan and participate in fire safety classes and evacuation drills.

Effective fire safety measures also include:

1. Smoking only in designated smoking areas
2. Fire inspections that try to uncover potential fire hazards before they cause fires
3. Annual preventative maintenance inspections on the heating and cooling units and other major electrical appliances/equipment
4. Installing smoke detectors and posting fire evacuation routes and fire exit signs
5. Regular checks on smoke detectors and fire extinguishers
6. Health care workers who are constantly alert to potential fire hazards

Electrical Safety

Electrical safety involves proper use of electrical equipment and basic maintenance of the cords and circuits. Electrical equipment should be located away from sinks and other water reservoirs to avoid the possibility of electric shock. Electrical cords should be routinely inspected and broken or frayed cords replaced. Extension cords are a potential hazard and should not be overloaded with multiple appliances connected. Electric cords should not be draped around other items. A three-prong or safety plug provides added electrical grounding and is generally provided with heavy duty equipment or equipment that is in constant use, such as the electrocardiograph and laboratory centrifuge machines.

Accidents

Accidents do not just happen, they result from someone's inattention to details. Common sources of accidents are:

- Loose area rugs or torn carpet
- Unstable furniture or broken furniture
- Dangling electrical cords
- Young children or confused/disoriented person left alone/unattended
- Wet floors or highly waxed floors

The key to avoiding accidents is prevention. Each health worker should carefully look at his/her work environment and reduce or eliminate potential accident conditions.

Reporting Accidents. Accidents should be reported immediately to the staff supervisor. Each medical facility will have a procedure for reporting and recording accidents. Remember prevention is better than a cure. **Refer to Task 4-3 in the appendix, Preparing Safety Reports (Accident/ Incident).**

PRINCIPLES OF BODY MECHANICS

Health workers use physical effort to perform their jobs. Injury and fatigue are less likely to occur if proper body mechanics are used. Also, by applying the principles of body mechanics, limited radiographers can prevent patient injuries resulting from improper lifting and moving.

The term "body mechanics" refers to good posture, alignment of the body segments, and correct use of muscles or muscle groups. Good posture occurs when all parts of the body are in balance and each segment aligned, Figure 4-4. Good posture provides a balanced body that is steady and secure and less prone to improper muscle use, falls, and mishaps. In addition to a balanced stable body, good posture allows the internal organs to work with greater efficiency. The following are tips for good posture:

1. Stand with feet parallel and four to eight inches apart.
2. Keep body weight equally distributed on both feet.
3. Hold head erect with chin held in.
4. Hold chest and shoulders up.
5. Keep knees slightly bent.

Good posture needs to be maintained during the performance of workday activities. Basic tips for good body mechanics during task performance are:

■ Keep the body's line close to the center of gravity (the waistline) when moving or lifting patients or objects.
■ Bend the knees when picking up an object from the floor. Do not bend from the waist.

Figure 4-4. Correct posture, upright position. In the upright position, the center of gravity is the center of the pelvis.

■ Pull weight with the upper arms using the biceps.

■ Balance the load over both feet when lifting. Bring the patient or object close to the body, bend the knees, and set the spine to support the load. Use arm muscles to lift. Always keep body balanced. Do not twist the body to move with a load, rather change foot positions.

■ Keep body balanced over feet and spread feet apart to provide a base of support.

MOVING AND TRANSPORTING PATIENTS

Limited radiographers work in a variety of settings and will encounter all kinds of patients. Examples of patient types follow.

Ambulatory patients—those who can walk and move. Ambulatory patients may require aides such as a walker, cane, or crutches.

Nonambulatory patients—those who cannot walk and move. Nonambulatory patients may arrive at the health care facility in an ambulance and be transported on a stretcher or a wheelchair. Ambulatory patients whose condition warrants may require transfer by wheelchair.

Before moving and transporting a patient, the radiographer must evaluate the patient's ability to aid in the process. Every patient must be considered in this evaluation since a patient's condition can change quickly. Generally, limited radiographers move and transport patients between a reception area or examination room to the radiography room and on and off the radiographic table. The following should be considered when assessing the patient:

■ *General condition*. How does the patient appear? Is the patient alert, responsive, oriented, and functioning?

■ *Mobility.* Did the patient walk into the facility without assistance? Are the patient's motions restricted in any way?

■ *Strength and endurance.* Can the patient stand and walk without assistance? If so, will the patient become fatigued and be unable to complete the transfer without resting or assistance?

■ *Balance.* Can the patient maintain balance? If the radiography procedure requires prolonged sitting or standing can the patient maintain the position without assistance?

■ *Understanding and acceptance.* Does the patient understand the need to move and be transported? Does the patient seem willing and accepting of the move and transfer, or is the patient fearful?

After the initial assessment, the limited radiographer must decide what is the best way to move the patient and how much help will be required to safely make the move and transport. Never attempt to move or transport a patient without adequate assistance; to do so may cause injury to self or patient. It is helpful to remember the following rules related to patient transport:

■ Move and transfer a patient over the shortest distance.
■ Inform the patient about the move and ask for cooperation and help.
■ Give short, simple commands.
■ Give only the help the patient needs for safety and comfort.
■ For standing and walking transfers, the patient should wear shoes.
■ Lock all wheels on stretchers and wheelchairs before assisting the patient to move.

Methods of Transfer

Patient transfer can be divided into ambulatory and nonambulatory methods and the skills and safety precautions associated with each.

Although a patient is ambulatory, an initial assessment should be conducted. It is the limited radiographer's responsibility to remain alert and observant of any change in status of the ambulatory patient and give assistance as needed.

The ambulatory patient should be provided with a footstool when getting on and off the radiography table. Also, it is best to walk with the ambulatory patient instead of way ahead or behind, just in case assistance is required.

In transferring nonambulatory patients, the limited radiographer must take great care to prevent further injury and to protect the skin. These patients may be handicapped, paralyzed, seriously injured, and/or unconscious. The body, head, and neck will require support during the move. Common methods of transfer include using a three-carrier lift, sheet transfer, and logrolling the patient. **Refer to Task 4-4 in the appendix for the procedure for using a three-carrier lift, to Task 4-5 for the procedure for transferring a patient using a sheet, and to Task 4-6 for the procedure for logrolling the patient.**

Patients may use a walking aid to support their body. Patients with walking aids will require the greatest assistance when moving through heavy doors, narrow hallways, and especially in small dressing areas and in getting on and off the radiographic table.

Canes are used to provide balance and support when there is a weakness on one side of the body. A walker provides more support than a cane because it has four points of support. Limited radiographers should be alert to potential falls and loss of balance in the patient with a cane or walker. Should such an incident occur, the limited radiographer should provide support to the patient's weak side until s/he has regained support and balance on the cane or walker.

Crutches are used when one lower extremity is injured or when both extremities need strength. Patients with crutches are always at risk of falling because they must rest the upper arm weight on the crutches. When assisting the patient with crutches on and off the radiographic table, it is best to seek assistance and have support on both sides of the patient. **Refer to Task 4-7 in the appendix for the procedure for assisting the patient with an ambulatory aid: cane, walker, and crutches. Also refer to the following tasks in the appendix:**

Task 4-8 Transporting the Patient in a Wheelchair
Task 4-9 Transferring the Patient between Radiographic Table and Wheelchair

THE PATIENT'S RECORD: A RESOURCE DOCUMENT

Health care agencies use many types of forms for recording information about a patient. All of the forms used for a patient are placed in a folder and make up the patient's record. Charting is the process of making entries on the patient's record.

The patient's records serve many purposes:

- Guide to planning patient care
- Source of shared information that promotes continuity of the patient's care
- Source of information to keep all health personnel informed about the patient's care and condition
- Permanent summary of the patient's health status
- Research statistics
- Legal document

Making Entries on Patient Records

Each medical facility has certain guidelines about making entries on a patient's record. Such guidelines include who is responsible for writing on each form, the type of charting notations made, and what forms become part of the patient's permanent record.

Limited radiographers use patient records and make entries related to radiography procedures and basic patient care. Since limited radiographers generally function as a multiskilled professional, there may be many opportunities to refer to a patient's record and to make entries. Some examples are:

■ The limited radiographer escorts a patient to the examination room, asks for the chief complaint, measures and records the vital signs, and enters the measurements on the patient record.
■ The limited radiographer receives an oral telephone report on a special radiography procedure performed by a referral agency. The report is recorded and becomes part of the patient's record.
■ The limited radiographer checks the chart to confirm the doctor's oral request for a radiograph.

Table 4-1 gives suggestions for making entries on a patient's medical record.

TABLE 4–1 MAKING ENTRIES ON PATIENT MEDICAL RECORD

SUGGESTION	EXPLANATION
Use a pen to make entries.	The patient's record is a legal document and entries made in pencil can be too easily erased.
Make legible entries.	Write or print so others may read the penmanship. Illegible entries are useless.
Enter month, day, year.	Entries not properly dated lose their value as a source of information exchange and as a legal document. Many medical facilities also enter the time of day and A.M. or P.M.

TABLE 4–1   (CONTINUED)

SUGGESTION	EXPLANATION
Follow facility policy concerning what should be recorded.	It is not necessary to record everything, follow facility policy.
Be brief and concise.	■ Omit *a*, *an*, and, *the*. ■ Omit writing patient name. ■ Use only standard common medical abbreviations.
Avoid personal judgment statements such as "seems like" or "appears to be." Quote the patient whenever possible. Record any adverse reactions, incidents, or mishaps the patient has.	If adverse reactions or unusual incidents are not recorded, it can be assumed they were not present. If the procedure or treatment requests are not documented as being carried out, it can be assumed they were not.
Some facilities require that documentation be made when ordered tests and procedures are completed. Describe instructions that a patient receives about examination preparation or self-administered contrast media. Do not rely on memory — record promptly.	Errors and omissions are likely if you rely on memory only.
Draw a line through an area left blank when not filled with information. Do not use ditto marks. Do not erase. Draw a single line through the error, write "error" near. Sign or initial all entries. Do not record for another person.	The line indicates that the area left blank was not intentionally omitted. Also, erasures may suggest falsification of information or facts.

MEETING PATIENTS' NEEDS

During any given day, a limited radiographer will provide care to a number of patients, each with a specific radiographic examination need. To complete the radiographs requested, patients may require assistance with meeting general and personal needs. Information related to meeting general and personal patient needs follows.

Physical Needs

Be aware of and provide for patients' privacy while they are dressing and undressing. Do not insist on staying with patients unless they ask for assistance or appear unable to help themselves. Knock on closed doors before entering, and close doors during procedures.

Limited radiographers may not notice how cool the room temperature feels because they are busy working; however, to the patient who may be disrobed, the room may be very cool. Provide a light blanket or sheet for the patient to use if s/he feels chilled.

Other Needs

Patient valuables, such as a purse, wallet, watch, jewelry, eyeglasses, dentures, prostheses, or other such items, should never be left unattended. Ask patients to keep these items with them at all times. If a patient's valuables are stolen, report this immediately to the supervisor.

Patients may need assistance in finding or ambulating to the bathroom. Bathrooms should be kept stocked at all times with adequate toilet paper, paper towels, soap, and sanitary pads. Patients who cannot ambulate to the bathroom, may require assistance or a urinal or a bedpan. Limited radiographers may require additional assistance in positioning a patient on a bedpan.

IV TUBES, URINARY CATHETERS, NASAL OXYGEN

Patients who have connecting IV tubes, urinary catheters, or nasal oxygen should be moved with care so as to not disturb these items. The limited radiographer's task is to take the required radiographs and to be observant of these items. If the IV tubing or urinary catheter becomes disconnected, it is important to report this immediately to the attending supervisor.

Limited radiographers often encounter patients who are receiving oxygen therapy. Without an adequate supply of oxygen in the body, metabolic activity decreases and life processes end. When individuals are unable to maintain a sufficient level of oxygen within their bodies, devices must be used to supplement their oxygen. It is safe to say that persons who require oxygen therapy are seriously ill and must be attended to carefully. An extremely important fact to remember is that *oxygen has properties that support combustion* and therefore becomes dangerous in the presence of sparks or flames. Although limited radiographers *do not* administer any type of oxygen therapy, it is important to recognize proper handling of patients receiving oxygen. Because oxygen is a highly combustible gas and radiographic equipment can cause sparks, the limited radiographer must always be extremely cautious and reduce the possibility of static electricity sparks when working where oxygen is being administered. Smoking is not allowed when oxygen is in use.

The amount of oxygen a patient is to receive is ordered by a physician. The various types of therapy devices are: (1) *nasal cannula*, (2) *nasal catheter*, (3) *face mask*, and (4) *oxygen tent*.

If an oxygen nasal cannula or face mask becomes dislodged or disconnected from the patient, the limited radiographer should put the nasal cannula or face mask back in place and ask the supervisor to check the equipment and the oxygen supply.

In most busy institutions where oxygen therapy is administered, experienced personnel are available to operate equipment and to provide assistance as needed.

VITAL SIGNS

Limited radiographers must have knowledge of and be able to measure a patient's *vital signs*, i.e., those measures that let us know how a patient is doing on very basic levels of functioning—body temperature, pulse rate, blood pressure, and respiration rate. It is very important for limited radiographers to know the normal ranges of vital signs so that they can recognize deviations from the normal, which often indicate a medical emergency.

The definition of a medical emergency is a sudden, unexpected change in a person's vital functions that demands immediate action. In the medical setting, emergencies may not be unexpected if the patient has had appropriate clinical assessment and is receiving medical treatment. Accordingly, there may be signs that all medical personnel who come in contact with the patient should recognize—signs that indicate trouble or a change in the patient's condition. For example, a patient's lips turning blue is a sign of a serious loss of oxygen to the brain and requires immediate action. *Immediate action* is probably the most critical aspect of any emergency; it is the required spontaneous reaction to the situation that actually constitutes the emergency.

Vital signs are important and useful because they provide the first signs of trouble for a patient; they also gauge a patient's return to a stable condition following physiological disturbances.

Temperature

Temperature is the expressed heat or coldness of the body as measured by a scaled thermometer. The normal or average body temperature registered by a healthy person is 98.6° F or 37° C. Average temperature may vary one to two degrees above or below 98.6° F and still be within normal limits. It is very important that a person's normal temperature be kept regulated.

A high temperature is called a fever or febrile, and if it is allowed to remain high (i.e., four or five degrees above 98.6° F) too long, damage to the central nervous system cells may result. The physician's orders must always be followed to reduce the patient's fever.

Three methods used for taking temperature are: (1) oral, (2) rectal, and (3) axillary. Temperatures may be measured by a mercury thermometer or an electronic (battery-operated) thermometer, Figures 4-5 and 4-6.

To take a temperature orally, use an oral, glass tube, clinical thermometer with an elongated tip. Before placing a thermometer in the patient's mouth, clean the thermometer and shake the mercury down until it registers 96° F

Figure 4-5. Clinical thermometers. *Top to bottom:* oral, security, rectal. These thermometers use the Fahrenheit scale of temperature measurement. *(From Hegner & Caldwell.* Nursing Assistant, A Nursing Process Approach. *6th ed. Delmar Publishers Inc., 1992. ISBN 4800-2. Figure 14-5, p. 229.)*

or below. The thermometer should be placed under the tongue for three to five minutes with the patient's mouth closed. If the patient has just ingested hot or cold liquids or foods or has just smoked, wait fifteen to thirty minutes before taking the oral temperature. **Refer to Task 4-11 in the appendix for the procedure for taking temperature using mercury and electronic thermometers.**

Use an oral thermometer to take axillary (under the arm) temperature. Leave the thermometer in place for ten minutes in a dry armpit. This is the least reliable measure of temperature and generally is one degree lower than oral measurement.

To take temperature rectally, use a blunt tip (short, rounded) glass thermometer made specifically for rectal temperature measurement. This method is generally used on children or on adults whenever oral readings are uncertain. The thermometer is lubricated and placed within the rectum about one and one-half inches; it must be held in place two to three minutes. Red protective cover sheaths may be available to cover the thermometer. The temperature is generally one degree above oral measurement.

Figure 4-6. An electronic thermometer. The temperature is registered in large, easy-to-read numerals. The disposable protective sheath is placed over the probe tip. The probe is then placed in the patient's mouth in the usual manner. *(Courtesy IVAC Corporation)*

Pulse

Each beat of the heart is a pulsation that occurs when the heart contracts (tightens) to send blood through the arterial system. The beat or pulse may be felt at certain places on the body starting at the head and moving downward to the feet, Figure 4-7. The name and location of the different pulses are:

- *Temporal*—in front of the ear at the temple
- *Carotid*—in the front of the neck over the carotid artery
- *Apical*—actual heartbeat over apex of the heart; heard with a stethoscope
- *Brachial*—over the brachial artery at the inner surface of the elbow

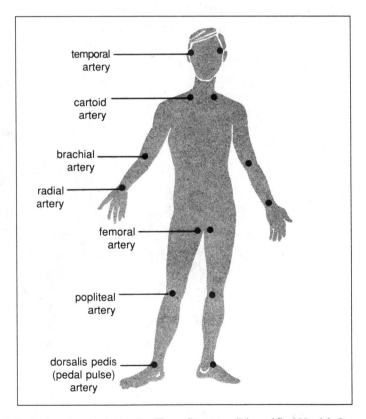

Figure 4-7. Pulse sites in the body. *(From Simmers*, Diversified Health Occupations, *1988, Delmar Publishers Inc.) (From Hegner & Caldwell.* Nursing Assistant, A Nursing Process Approach. *6th ed. Delmar Publishers Inc., 1992. ISBN 4800-2. Figure 15-1, p. 242.)*

- *Radial*—at the wrist just above the base of the thumb
- *Femoral*—in the groin over the femoral artery
- *Popliteal*—posterior or just behind the knee joint
- *Pedal*—on the arch of the foot at the dorsal pedal (dorsalis pedis) artery

The most common areas used to check pulse rate are (a) apical, with a stethoscope for accurate rate, and (b) radial, with the first two fingers placed on the inner side of the wrist at the depression just above the thumb. The farther away from the heart the pulse rate is taken, the more difficult it becomes to count because the pulse wave weakens.

Normal *pulse rates* range from fifty to one hundred beats per minute for adults. Many activities and events will cause a change in the heart rate, thus resulting in a change in the pulse rate. Table 4-2 shows average pulse beats per minute according to age groups. Pulse rates are affected by age, body build, exercise, medications (drugs), blood pressure, body temperature, pain, and various foods and liquids.

There are several aspects to consider when checking pulse rates. A *regular* pulse has constant rhythm and equal time between pulses; this indicates good blood flow. An *irregular* pulse has inconsistent rhythm and may be felt as both strong and weak throbs. A *thready* pulse is weak, difficult to count, and irregular in rhythm; this pulse indicates poor blood flow. As stated earlier, when you are counting the radial pulse, place the tips of your first two fingers over the radial artery of the patient's wrist at the inner portion of the wrist just above the thumb and count the pulse beats for one minute. Do not apply your own thumb to the patient's wrist because the thumb has its own strong pulse. The procedure for pulse count is included

TABLE 4–2   AVERAGE PULSE BEATS PER MINUTE ACCORDING TO AGE GROUPS

		2 Years	4 Years	6 Years	8 Years	10 Years	12 Years	16 Years
	PULSE RATE PER MINUTE							
	Newborn							
Female	115–130	110	100	100	90	90	90	90
Male	115–130	110	100	100	90	90	85	75

with the procedure for counting respiration because pulse and respiration are generally checked together. **Refer to Task 4-12 in the appendix for the procedure for counting the radial pulse and the respiratory rate.**

Respiration

The exchange of oxygen and carbon dioxide in the lungs is called respiration. Respiration occurs when a person takes in a breath (inhales) and lets out a breath (exhales). One such exchange is counted as one excursion of breathing. This exchange of gases is done at the rate of sixteen to twenty times a minute by the average adult.

Changes that occur in the chest during inhalation and exhalation are important considerations for the limited radiographer when doing a chest film. During chest radiography, it is important that the limited radiographer allow the patient to breathe in and out a couple of times to ensure that the lungs are fully inflated and that the diaphragm has moved down, allowing more lung to be visualized.

To reduce possible patient anxiety, it is best to count respirations when the patient is unaware that the count is being taken. The rate of breathing, like pulse, can be affected by such common considerations as age (children breathe faster, older people slower), exercise, emotions, disease, temperature, and medications.

Respirations may be counted after a patient's pulse has been taken. To do so, it is best to continue holding the wrist so the patient will not realize you are counting breathing excursions (inhalations and exhalations). To count respiration, count the number of times the patient's chest moves up or rises. Count respirations for sixty seconds. When observing a child, breathe with the child; this technique is particularly useful when you are making a radiographic exposure of the chest on full inhalation. It is equally important to listen to the patient's breathing to determine if it is labored or unusual in sound. Normal breathing should be relaxed, even and quiet. Respiration should be recorded as *regular, irregular, rapid, shallow,* or *labored*. Table 4-3 lists the medical term given to abnormal types of breathing and the characteristics of each.

Blood Pressure

Blood pressure (BP) is the force of the flow of blood exerted against the walls of the blood vessels. Blood pressure is measured by reading two num-

TABLE 4–3 ABNORMAL TYPES OF BREATHING AND CHARACTERISTICS OF EACH TYPE	
Apnea	Temporary cessation of breathing; suspended respiration.
Cheyne-Stokes	Bizarre breathing where apnea occurs from ten to sixty seconds followed by increased depth and frequency of breathing.
Dyspnea	Audible labored or difficult breathing.
Hyperventilation	Increased respiratory rate or breathing that is deeper than normal; forced respiration.
Rales	Abnormal sounds heard in the chest, caused by air passage in the bronchi that contains secretion.
Rapid breathing	An increase in respiration rate; as in hyperventilation.
Shallow breathing	A type of breathing that occurs in acute pulmonary disease when chest walls are thick.
Stridor	Obstructed air passages that create a harsh sound during respiration; high-pitched sound like wind blowing.
Wheeze	Whistling sound as a result of narrowing of the lumen of respiratory passageway.

bers that register on an aneroid or mercury gauge called a sphygmomanometer, Figure 4-8.

Two numbers are read for blood pressure: (1) when the heart contracts or *systolic* pressure and (2) when the heart is relaxed or *diastolic* pressure.

Figure 4-8. Aneroid manometer-type of sphygmomanometer for measuring blood pressure. Different size cuffs are shown. For an accurate measurement of blood pressure, it is important to use the proper size cuff on the patient. For example, a large adult cuff should not be used on a child. *(From Hegner & Caldwell.* Nursing Assistant, A Nursing Process Approach. *6th ed. Delmar Publishers Inc., 1992. ISBN 4800-2. Figure 16-3, p. 248.)*

The average adult's blood pressure should be 120/80 mm of mercury. The top number (120) is the systolic pressure and the bottom number (80) is the diastolic pressure. Blood pressure is crucial to good health and may be affected by many things.

The same activities and events that affect the pulse also affect blood pressure. Other important situations prevalent in our society today that cause blood pressure problems are (1) heart and kidney disease, (2) vascular disease in the brain, (3) emotional conditions, (4) drugs, and (5) higher blood pressure in men than women in the same age group.

Hypertension and hypotension are two conditions with which the health professional needs to be familiar. *Hypertension* is high blood pressure created and exacerbated (made worse) by a variety of conditions including disease, emotional stress, and environmental stress. *Hypotension* is low blood pressure and is not necessarily an indication of illness unless the person has symptoms. However, low blood pressure related to shock or circulatory collapse is dangerous and can result in death if not treated.

To ensure accurate readings, these rules must be followed:

1. Select the appropriate cuff size to fit the patient.
2. Inflate and deflate the cuff gradually.
3. Palpate the pulse before placing the stethoscope firmly over the brachial artery.
4. Ask the patient to be absolutely still.

Table 4-4 shows average blood pressures for age groups according to sex. Blood pressure will vary with age and physical condition. **Refer to Task 4-13 in the appendix for the procedure for taking blood pressure.**

MEDICAL EMERGENCIES

Medical emergencies can and do occur in the office radiography environment. The limited radiographer must therefore have basic knowledge about medical emergencies and the immediate actions required.

Fainting

Fainting is probably the most common emergency that occurs in the radiography setting. The limited radiographer must constantly observe all patients for signs of dizziness, pallor, or cold, clammy skin. At the first sign of fainting, have the patient lie down or place the head between the legs lower than the body. Application of cool compresses on the face may also be effective. Seek assistance as soon as possible.

TABLE 4–4 AVERAGE BLOOD PRESSURE ACCORDING TO AGE GROUPS

		BP MM HG						
	Newborn	2 Years	4 Years	6 Years	8 Years	10 Years	12 Years	16 Years
Female		98/60	98/60	98/64	104/68	110/72	114/74	120/78
Male		96/60	96/60	98/62	102/68	110/72	112/74	124/78

Seizures

Seizures are caused by medical problems ranging from emotion or anxiety reactions to brain tumors. Epilepsy, usually found in children or young adults, is probably the most common cause of seizures. The most important response to a seizure is to make sure that the patient does not injure his/her head or body during the convulsive phase or obstruct his/her airway with his/her tongue. It is best to simply stay with the patient and call for assistance.

A mild seizure (petit mal) may be of short duration or may go unnoticed. A more severe seizure (grand mal) always requires assistance. Some symptoms of grand mal are jerky movements, rapid breathing, a loud cry, muscle rigidity, incontinence of urine or stool, vomiting, and frothing (foaming at the mouth). All symptoms that occur before, during, and after a seizure should be reported to a supervisor. The limited radiographer should make no attempt to open the patient's mouth or to force a solid object (such as wrapped tongue blades) into the mouth or airway.

Nosebleeds

Bleeding or hemorrhage from the nose is usually referred to as epistaxis. *Universal Blood and Body Fluid Precautions* should be used when attempting to control bleeding. Nosebleeds may be controlled by applying external pressure to the side of the bleeding nostril. Cold compresses to the face may also be of value. The patient's head should be elevated. Seek assistance from the supervisor or attending physician.

REVIEW QUESTIONS

1. Select the correct statements regarding nosocomial infections by placing a check mark (✔) beside the statement. A nosocomial infection
   _____ is generally acquired in hospitals or medical care settings
   _____ is more common in healthy adults
   _____ is considered opportunistic
   _____ can be reduced by using common asepsis
2. Asepsis is defined as the (circle the letter of the correct response)
   a) absence of all disease-producing organisms
   b) reduction of most disease-producing organisms

3. Match the following terms to the correct statement.

_____ Surgical asepsis   a) reduction of microorganisms by using chemical methods

_____ Disinfection   b) absence of all disease-producing organisms

_____ Asepsis   c) procedures used to destroy microorganisms before they enter the body

4. Select the correct statement regarding the following. The Centers for Disease Control recommends using universal precautions with (check one)

_____ a) patients who appear ill

_____ b) patients who have been diagnosed as HIV carriers

_____ c) all patients regardless of their appearance or diagnosis

5. Normal adult body temperature when taken orally is (check one)

_____ a) 96.6°F

_____ b) 99.6°F

_____ c) 97.6°F

_____ d) 98.6°F

6. Normal adult pulse rate is within the range of (check one)

_____ a) 50–70

_____ b) 30–40

_____ c) 50–100

_____ d) 115–130

7. Normal adult blood pressure range is (check one)

_____ a) 110/140

_____ b) 120/80

_____ c) 90/110

_____ d) 70/80

8. Most people are free of infection most of the time because (check one)

_____ a) there are few disease-causing organisms in the environment

_____ b) microorganisms gain entrance to the body only through a break in the skin

_____ c) microorganisms do not adhere to the skin of the body

_____ d) the body's defense mechanisms protect it from invading germs

REFERENCES

1. *Morbidity and Mortality Weekly Report*. Centers for Disease Control. August 21, 1987, Vol. 36, No. 25. U.S. Department of Health and Human Services, Atlanta, GA.

2. "Update: Universal Precautions for Prevention of Transmission of Human Immunodeficiency Virus, Hepatitis B Virus, and Other Bloodborne Pathogens in Health-Care Settings," *Morbidity and Mortality Weekly Report, Supplement.* Centers for Disease Control. June 24, 1988, Vol. 37, No. 24, pp. 377–82, 387–88. U.S. Department of Health and Human Services, Atlanta, GA.

3. Torres, Lillian S., and Carol Morrill. *Basic Medical Techniques and Patient Care for Radiologic Technologists.* 2d ed. Philadelphia: J.B. Lippincott Company, 1983.

BIBLIOGRAPHY

Answers About AIDS. A Report by the American Council on Science and Health. New York: American Council on Science and Health, 1988.

Cooper, Marian G., and David E. Cooper. *The Medical Assistant.* 5th ed. New York: McGraw-Hill Book Company, 1986.

Ehrlich, Ruth A., and Ellen M. Givens. *Patient Care in Radiology.* 2d ed. St. Louis: The C. V. Mosby Company, 1985.

Miller, Benjamin F., and Clair B. Keane. *Encyclopedia and Dictionary of Medicine, Nursing, and Allied Health.* Philadelphia: W. B. Saunders Company, 1987.

Rambo, Beverly J., and L. A. Wood. *Nursing Skills for Clinical Practice.* Philadelphia: W. B. Saunders Company, 1982.

Thomas, Clayton L. (Ed.). *Taber's Cyclopedic Medical Dictionary.* 15th ed. Philadelphia: F. A. Davis, 1985.

CHAPTER

5

Radiographic Physics

CHAPTER OUTLINE

OBJECTIVES

Upon completion of the chapter, the student will demonstrate knowledge, facts, and principles presented through oral and written evaluation.

1. Identify the common units of measurement and atomic nomenclature.
2. Label an atomic illustration with the following energy shells: nucleus, proton, electron, neutron.
3. State the electric charge of a neutron, electron, and proton.
4. Draw an illustration showing atomic structure before and after ionization of the atom.
5. Identify the smallest unit of an atom, element, and compound.
6. List the origin and characteristics of electromagnetic radiation (gamma rays and X rays) and particulate radiation.

7. Identify the definition for the electrostatics and magnetism terminology list.
8. Match common electricity and magnetism laws and principles to their definition or application example.

"Why must I study physics?" and "How does physics relate to the everyday job of medical radiography?" are common questions asked by radiography students. Such questions express the students' need to understand how physics and related concepts apply to the everyday tasks performed by medical radiographers. One answer to these questions is that the basic laws and concepts of physics form the foundation of X-ray production, X-ray interaction, and radiographic image formation.

This chapter presents the essential laws and concepts of physics that have a direct application to medical radiography.

Part I:
Natural Science Review

INTRODUCTION

Physics is a branch of science that deals with matter and energy and their relation to each other. It includes heat, sound, light, mechanics, electricity, magnetism, and the basic structure and properties of matter. Physics, like chemistry, astronomy, and geology, is considered one of the physical sciences and is classified as a natural science.

UNITS OF MEASUREMENT

Because physics is a science, it needs a way to accurately describe the physical reality with which it deals. This is accomplished with a system of measurement to describe physical quantities such as length, mass, or time. In the United States, the common measurement system uses units such as inches, feet, quarts, or pounds. The rest of the world, especially the scientific world, uses the International System of Units (SI units). These units are based on the familiar metric system where the meter is the standard of length, the kilogram is the standard of mass, and the second is the standard of time. All other SI units are derived from these few base units and are used to describe such quantities as area (square meters), velocity (meters/second), or volume (cubic meters). Other SI units based on more complex combinations of the base units are given special names such as the unit of force (the newton) or the unit of energy (the joule). The quantities of the units represented may be modified by the use of suitable prefixes. For example, a kilometer is 1000 meters and a millisecond is 1/1000 of a second. Table 5-1 presents the base units, some of the derived units common to radiology and their special names, and the meaning of the prefixes used to modify the units.

CONCEPTS OF MATTER

The universe consists of matter and energy. Matter may be defined in terms of its properties such as mass or volume. **Energy** is the ability to do work, where work is defined as the application of force over a distance. There are many different forms of energy, such as mechanical, electrical, or heat. There are two types of the various forms of energy: kinetic and potential.

Kinetic energy is energy of motion. When an object is moving, it possesses kinetic energy. Examples of kinetic energy are a pitched baseball, a moving automobile, or a person walking. Because any moving object possesses two quantities, mass and velocity, kinetic energy is expressed in terms of mass and velocity.

Potential energy is stored energy. Potential energy exists because of an object's position. For this reason, it is called energy of position. On the earth, an object's potential energy depends on its height above the ground. Any object may possess either kinetic energy or potential energy or both. For example, if a person holds a ball above the ground, it will have potential energy by virtue of its height. However, it will have zero kinetic energy because it is not moving. If the ball is dropped and is falling, it will possess kinetic energy because of its motion and it will also have potential energy because it is still above the ground. At the instant the ball strikes the ground, the kinetic energy will be at its maximum while the potential energy will be zero.

TABLE 5–1   SYSTEMS OF MEASUREMENT

British System	Foot, pound, second
Metric System	Centimeter, gram, second, meter, kilogram
SI System (International System of Units)	A new system of measurement in science that provides for the interconversion of units among all branches of science. Based on the metric system.
Units of Measurement	
Length	The unit of length. The *meter* (m) is the basic unit of length in the metric system.
Mass	A measurement of the quantity of matter in a body. The *kilogram* (kg) is the SI unit of mass.
Time	Measurement of intervals between events. The standard unit of time is *second*(s).
Area	Measurement of a given surface dependent upon length of area; square meters (m^2).
Volume	Measurement of the capacity of a container, dependent upon length of container. Volume may be expressed in cubic meters (m^3), liters (l), milliliters (ml), or cubic centimeters (cc or cm^3).
Velocity	Speed in a given direction. Expressed in meters per second (m/s).

Temperature	Expressed as degrees Celsius or Fahrenheit.
	 Celsius = 0°C freezing point of water
	           100°C boiling point of water
	 Fahrenheit = 32°F freezing point of water
	           212°F boiling point of water

The **Law of Conservation of Energy** states that energy can be neither created nor destroyed but can be changed into other forms of energy. Some different types of energy are mechanical, thermal, radiant, electrical, chemical, and nuclear, and change can occur between these forms. The change of energy from one form to another is called a transformation of energy. Table 5-2 gives examples of energy transformation.

While energy can exist in many different forms, matter exists in only three states: solid, liquid, and gas. Matter can be converted from one state to another, depending upon conditions of pressure and temperature. For example, water is a liquid form of matter. However, when it is subjected to freezing temperatures, the state of water is converted into a solid—ice. Heated to boiling, water becomes a gas in the form of steam. Matter can be in either a state of rest (inertia) or motion (momentum). Matter is described by the physical quantities associated with these states, such as mass, volume, or temperature.

All matter is composed of atoms. The **atom** is the smallest particle into which matter can be divided while still maintaining a unique identity. The identities of different types of matter are distinguished by how they react chemically. Atoms that have different chemistries are considered distinct **elements**. There are presently 109 separate elements. The atomic and chemical relationship of one element to another follows a regular pattern that is described by the **Periodic Table of Elements**, Figure 5-1. All elements in the same vertical column (group) have similar chemical reactions.

Atoms of the same or different elements may be chemically combined to form **molecules**. Molecules, which themselves have distinct physical properties, form the basis for the complex chemical substances called **compounds**.

TABLE 5–2 EXAMPLES OF ENERGY TRANSFORMATION	
Baking powder/yeast	Causes baking mixtures to rise.
Chemical battery	Converts to electrical energy to power a flashlight or radio.
Sunlight	Captured in photosensitive solar cells for conversion to electricity.

PERIODIC TABLE OF THE ELEMENTS

Legend:
- 6 — Atomic Number
- C — Element Symbol
- 12 — Atomic Mass Number

Group Period	I	II										III	IV	V	VI	VII	VIII
1	1 H 1																2 He 4
2	3 Li 7	4 Be 9										5 B 11	6 C 12	7 N 14	8 O 16	9 F 19	10 Ne 20
3	11 Na 23	12 Mg 24										13 Al 27	14 Si 28	15 P 31	16 S 32	17 Cl 36	18 A 40
4	19 K 39	20 Ca 40	21 Sc 45	22 Ti 48	23 V 51	24 Cr 52	25 Mn 55	26 Fe 56	27 Co 59	28 Ni 59	29 Cu 64	30 Zn 65	31 Ga 70	32 Ge 73	33 As 75	34 Se 79	35 Br 80	36 Kr 84
5	37 Rb 86	38 Sr 88	39 Y 89	40 Zr 91	41 Nb 93	42 Mo 96	43 Tc 99	44 Ru 101	45 Rh 103	46 Pd 106	47 Ag 108	48 Cd 112	49 In 115	50 Sn 119	51 Sb 122	52 Te 128	53 I 127	54 Xe 131
6	55 Cs 133	56 Ba 137	57 to 71	72 Hf 179	73 Ta 181	74 W 184	75 Re 186	76 Os 190	77 Ir 192	78 Pt 195	79 Au 197	80 Hg 201	81 Tl 204	82 Pb 207	83 Bi 209	84 Po 210	85 At 210	86 Rn 222
7	87 Fr 223	88 Ra 226	89 to 109															

Note: Elements 57 to 71 are the rare earth metals.

Elements 89 to 109 are the actinide metals.

Figure 5-1. Periodic Table of the Elements

For example, two atoms of hydrogen associate to form a molecule of hydrogen gas. When two atoms of hydrogen **associate**, or bond, with one atom of oxygen a molecule of water is formed, Figure 5-2. Many molecules of water form the compound water with which we are familiar and that may be described by such physical properties as its freezing point ($0°$ C, $32°$ F) and boiling point ($100°$ C, $212°$ F).

ATOMIC STRUCTURE

The atom, the basis for the elements, is itself made up of separate particles. All atoms are composed of three fundamental particles: the proton, the neutron, and the electron. The **proton** and the **neutron** are found in the center of the atom, called the **nucleus**, and have approximately the same mass. The proton has one positive electrical charge and the neutron is uncharged. For each positively charged proton in the nucleus of an uncharged atom there is one negatively charged (and much less massive) **electron** outside the nucleus, Figure 5-3. Since the number of positive particles (protons) in an atom equals the number of negative particles (electrons), the atom as a whole exists in an uncharged, or neutral, state.

The number of protons in an atom is called the **atomic number** (abbreviated Z) and the number of protons plus neutrons is the **atomic mass number** (A). Atoms are arranged on the periodic table by order of increasing atomic numbers.

Electrons exist in discrete positions outside the nucleus. These positions are called **orbitals** and represent the amount of energy individual electrons possess. Just as atoms of individual elements are arranged in the periodic table according to their atomic structure, electrons are arranged in a systematic fashion around the nucleus of an atom. Electrons are bound to atoms by an amount of energy, called the **electron binding energy**, which varies according to the position of the electrons. Electrons closest to the nucleus

Atoms → Molecules → Compounds

Hydrogen + Hydrogen + Oxygen → Water Molecule → Water

$$H + H + O \rightarrow H_2O \rightarrow H_2O + H_2O$$

Figure 5-2. Formation of a molecule of water

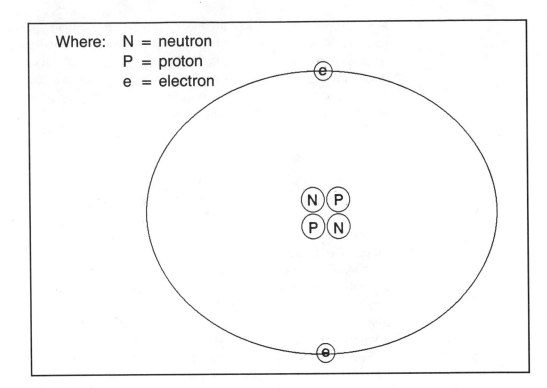

Figure 5-3. A simplified model of a helium atom

have the most binding energy and those farthest away the least. The orbitals in which the electrons are bound represent different energy levels. Each energy level, or shell, is designated by a different letter of the alphabet, beginning with the K-shell, closest to the nucleus, and proceeding through the L-, M-, N-, O-, P-, and Q-shells outward from the nucleus, Figure 5-4.

The numbers of electrons that can occupy each shell also follow a set of rules. If each electron shell is given a number starting with one for the K-shell, two for the L-shell, and so on, the maximum number of electrons that can fill that shell is given by the formula

$$2n^2 \text{ (2n(squared))}$$

Where: n is the number of the electron shell. Therefore, only two electrons are allowed in the K-shell, eight in the L-shell, and up to ninety-eight in the Q-shell. Another rule states that the maximum number of electrons allowed in the outer shell is eight.

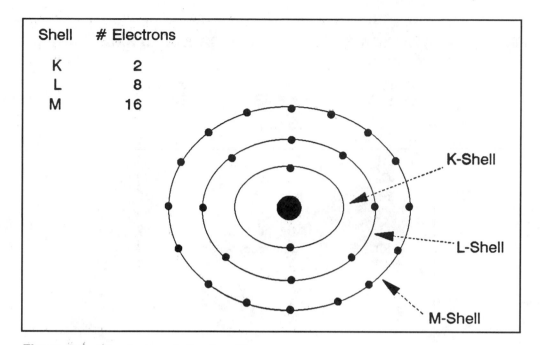

Shell	# Electrons
K	2
L	8
M	16

Figure 5-4. The electron shells of a sulfur atom

The number of electrons in the outer shell is related to the position of an element on the periodic table, with the number of outer shell electrons increasing from left to right. As it is the outer-shell electrons that determine the chemical reactivity of an atom, elements that react similarly are found in the same vertical column of the periodic table.

ATOMIC NOMENCLATURE

Elements are commonly shown in an alphabetic abbreviation. This is the **chemical symbol** of the element as shown in Table 5-3. To further distinguish separate elements, the atomic number (the number of protons) is written as a subscript to the left of the chemical symbol and the atomic mass number is written as a superscript to the left of the chemical symbol, Figure 5-5.

Atoms of the same element may have different numbers of neutrons in the nucleus while maintaining the same chemical identity. Atoms that have the same number of protons but different numbers of neutrons are called **isotopes**. Hydrogen is the simplest element, with a nucleus of one proton and one orbital electron. A neutron can be added to the nucleus of hydrogen, thus

TABLE 5–3   ELEMENTS IMPORTANT TO RADIOLOGY

CHEMICAL SYMBOL	ELEMENT	ATOMIC NUMBER (Z)	ATOMIC MASS NUMBER (A)
C	Carbon	6	12
O	Oxygen	8	16
Al	Aluminum	13	27
Ca	Calcium	20	40
Fe	Iron	26	56
Cu	Copper	29	63
Mo	Molybdenum	42	98
Ru	Ruthenium	44	102
Ag	Silver	47	107
Sn	Tin	50	120
I	Iodine	53	127
Ba	Barium	56	138
W	Tungsten	74	184
Pb	Lead	82	208

Figure 5-5. Atomic symbol nomenclature

giving an atomic mass number of two (one proton + one neutron). This atom is called deuterium, Figure 5-6. Chemically it is the same as hydrogen because it has one proton and one electron, but atomically it is different (an isotope of hydrogen) because it has one neutron.

IONIZATION

Atoms are electrically neutral, their electric charge being zero, because the total number of protons is equal to the number of electrons in the orbital shells. An atom may become **ionized** if it gains or loses an electron. Any charged particle is an **ion**. The loss of an electron results in a net positive charge and the atom is termed a **cation**. The addition of an electron to an atom results in a net negative charge and the atom is called an **anion**. An

Figure 5-6. Two isotopes of hydrogen

electron may be removed from an atom by the addition of energy to the atom. When this happens the removed electron and the electron from which it is removed are called an ion pair, Figure 5-7.

Types of Ionizing Radiation

Ionization may occur by the addition of energy to an atom. This energy may be added as pure energy or as matter. Energy or matter of this type is called **radiation**. If the radiation is in the form of matter it is called **particulate radiation**. If the radiation is in the form of pure energy, that is, without mass and charge, it is **electromagnetic radiation**. Since either type of radiation is capable of ionizing atoms, this radiation is collectively called **ionizing radiation**, Table 5-4.

Particulate radiation may occur as any of the common subatomic particles or as ionized atoms. Two common types of particulate radiation are alpha particles and beta particles. **Alpha particles**, or alpha rays, are the nuclei of helium atoms, two protons and two neutrons, and therefore have a charge of +2. **Beta particles** (beta rays) are physically identical to electrons. Both alpha particles and beta particles have the ability to remove electrons from atoms, thus ionizing the atoms.

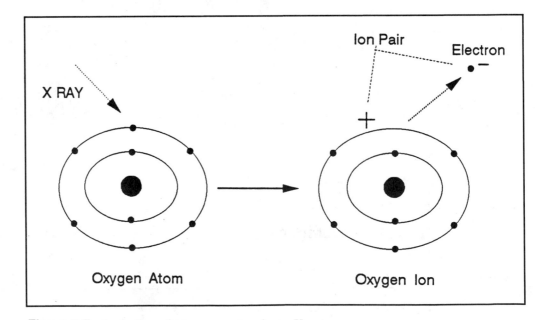

Figure 5-7. Ionization of an oxygen atom by an X ray

ELECTROMAGNETIC RADIATION

The matter of the universe exists in a sea of energy. Much of this energy is in the form of electromagnetic radiation. There are many types of electromagnetic radiation, such as visible light, radiowaves, or X rays. Electromagnetic radiation has no mass and no charge. It exists in the form of waves and may be described as a wave, Figure 5-8. If one considers the wave form in Figure 5-8, the distance from the peak of one wave to the next is the **wavelength** and is measured in meters. The height of a wave from the lowest valley to the highest peak is the **amplitude**. The part of a wave followed from halfway between a peak and valley up through the next peak and down

---

TABLE 5–4   IONIZING RADIATION

PARTICULATE

Subatomic particles in motion that originate from the nucleus of radioactive atoms. Radioactive atoms have nuclei that contain excess energy and particles. In an attempt to regain stability, these radioactive atoms emit their excess energy and particles.

RADIOACTIVE DECAY PROCESS

Alpha Particles	Beta Particles
(equivalent to two neutrons)	(equivalent to an electron)
can travel 5 cm	can travel 10–100 cm

Traveling particles of radiation

ELECTROMAGNETIC

Electromagnetic radiation differs from particulate in that it consists of bundles of energy (photons) and travels in wavelength form.

Two Types

Gamma radiation, like particulate radiation, originates from nucleus of radioactive atoms; however, it differs in that it exists as wavelengths of energy and is very penetrating to humans.

X ray is similar to gamma, but originates in orbitals.

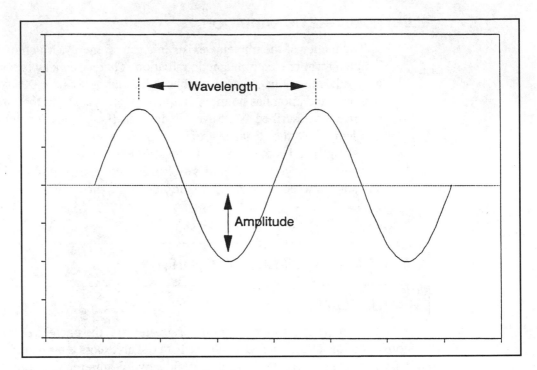

Figure 5-8. Amplitude and wavelength

through the next valley to the next midpoint is called one **cycle**. The number
of cycles passing through a given point in one second is the **frequency**. The
frequency is measured in cycles/second, given the name Hertz in SI units,
and abbreviated Hz.

Electromagnetic radiation is described by the three quantities of wavelength, frequency, and energy. The entire energy-frequency-wavelength range
of electromagnetic radiation is known as the **electromagnetic spectrum**,
Figure 5-9.

As may be seen from Figure 5-9, there are many different types of electromagnetic radiation. Visible light, to which the human eye responds, is inter-
mediate on the electromagnetic spectrum in energy. Just below visible light
are infrared radiation, which some insects can see; microwaves, used in
cooking and communications; and radiowaves. Just above visible light is
ultraviolet radiation, responsible to some extent for human "sun-tanning."
Above ultraviolet, X rays and gamma rays are found. Gamma rays are iden-

Figure 5-9. The electromagnetic spectrum

tical to X rays in every respect except in how they are produced. The higher the energy of electromagnetic radiation is, the better it can penetrate matter. Thus, X rays are used to penetrate the human body for radiographic imaging.

The energy and frequency of electromagnetic radiation are directly related—that is, the higher the energy is, the higher the frequency is. Energy and frequency are inversely related to wavelength: the higher the energy or frequency is, the shorter the wavelength.

Electromagnetic radiation is not one continuous waveform but instead consists of separate packets of energy called **quanta** (singular quantum) or more commonly **photons**. A photon may be thought of as a massless, uncharged bundle of radiation that has properties of continuous waves. Therefore, X rays are commonly spoken of as photons or X-ray photons. Photons are always in motion and always travel at the same velocity in a vacuum—300 million meters/second (186,000 miles/second). Since visible light is a type of electromagnetic radiation, this velocity is called the **speed of light**.

Part II:
Electricity and Magnetism

INTRODUCTION

Electricity is a form of energy. As energy it has the ability to do work. The work electricity does in an X-ray machine is the production of electro-magnetic radiation in the form of X rays. To understand how this occurs, one must first know something of the basic nature of electricity and magnetism.

ELECTRICITY

All atoms and subatomic particles have either a presence or absence of electrical charge. Protons have a single positive charge, electrons have a single negative charge, and neutrons have no charge. Atoms may have no charge, be singly charged, or have more than one charge, as long as the charge is a whole number (integer). Electrical charges obey certain physical laws, the most important being that like charges repel each other and unlike charges attract each other. A proton will be repelled by another proton but will attract an electron.

When an object has an electrical charge, it is said to be electrified or statically charged. The phenomenon of charged objects is termed **electro-statics** or **static electricity**. Electrification results from either a deficiency or an excess of electrons and occurs when electrons move from one object to another, Figure 5-10. The amount of electrification is measured in a unit called the **coulomb (C)**, which represents 6.3×10^{18} electron charges. Posi-tive charges do not move except in special cases involving ionized atoms.

The study of moving electrical charges is called **electrodynamics**. The movement of electrical charges, or electrons, occurs from one atom to another along the outside of a conductor. A **conductor** is a material that allows the easy movement of electrons. Most metals, such as copper, are good conductors. Materials, such as rubber or plastic, which impede the flow of electrons, are called **insulators**, Figure 5-11.

Figure 5-10. Electrification

Figure 5-11. Typical electrical wire

Electrical charges possess potential energy because they have the ability to do work by virtue of the repulsion of like charges and the attraction of unlike charges. This potential of electrical charges to do work is called **electrical potential**. The difference in electrical potential between two points on an electrical conductor is called the **potential difference**. This is analogous to mechanical potential energy. An object positioned above the ground has more potential energy than the same object on the ground because of the difference in height, or gravitational energy. In the same fashion, electrons at one end of a conductor have the ability to do work because they are repelling each other.

If a conductor is connected to a source of electrons, such as one end of a battery, and is connected to the other end of the battery to form an electrical circuit, electrons will flow along the conductor and work will be done. The amount of work performed by moving electrical charges is measured in volts (V). Electrons moving through a conductor are called **current**, which is measured in amperes (A).

If a circuit is modified to resist the flow of electrons, work can be extracted from the circuit in various forms, such as heat or radiant energy. Electrical resistance is measured in ohms (Ω). An **ohm** is the amount of resistance overcome by one volt to cause one ampere to flow.

The product of current (amperes) and resistance (ohms) is volts. This equation is expressed as:

$$V = IR$$

Where: V = voltage in volts, I = current in amperes, and R = resistance in ohms. This is called **Ohm's law** and forms the basis for the study of electrical circuits.

The amount of work that electricity does over a given amount of time is called **power** and is measured in watts (W).

MAGNETISM

Magnetism is the ability of some material to attract iron or ironlike substances. The magnetic property of a substance is defined by the magnetic field it creates. The magnetic field is the zone of influence of the magnetic property and is concentrated at two points called the **magnetic poles**. The earth itself is a huge magnet which has its magnetic poles at the geographical north and south. In a similar fashion, the poles of all magnets are called the north and south poles. A basic law of magnetism states that like poles repel each other and unlike poles attract each other.

Magnets may be naturally occurring substances or may be created by passing an electrical current through a conductor. This type of electromagnet is important in the operation of X-radiation generating equipment and will be discussed further in chapter 7.

REVIEW QUESTIONS

1. In ionization
   a) an electron may be removed from an atom
   b) a proton may be removed from an atom
   c) a neutron may be removed from an atom
   d) two of the above

2. Which of the following is a particulate radiation?
   a) X ray
   b) beta ray
   c) gamma ray
   d) two of the above

3. Which of the following statements is FALSE?
   a) A neutron has no charge.
   b) A proton has a positive charge.
   c) A neutron has approximately the same mass as an electron.
   d) A neutron has approximately the same mass as a proton.

4. Compounds are composed of _____ and molecules are composed of _____ .
   a) atoms, molecules
   b) molecules, neutrons
   c) molecules, atoms
   d) nucleons, atoms

5. How many atoms are there in one molecule of H_2O?
   a) 1
   b) 2
   c) 3
   d) 4

6. The SI unit of mass is the
   a) gram
   b) kilogram
   c) meter
   d) pound

7. Compared to radiowaves, X rays and gamma rays have
   1) higher energy and longer wavelength
   2) higher energy and shorter wavelength
   3) higher frequency and shorter wavelength
     a) 1 and 2
     b) 1 and 3
     c) 2 and 3
     d) 1, 2, and 3

8. Electrification occurs because of
   a) the movement of protons
   b) the movement of neutrons
   c) the movement of electrons
   d) the movement of atoms

9. Electric charge is measured in
   a) amperes
   b) coulombs
   c) volts
   d) ohms

10. Amperage is a measure of
   a) current
   b) force
   c) resistance
   d) charge

BIBLIOGRAPHY

Bushong, Stewart C. *Radiologic Science for Technologists Physics, Biology, and Protection*, 4th ed. St. Louis: The C.V. Mosby Company, 1988.

Currey, Thomas S., James E. Dowdey, and Robert C. Murry. *Christensen's Physics of Diagnostic Radiologic*. Philadelphia: Lea & Febiger, 1990.

Selman, Joseph. *The Fundamentals of X-Ray and Radium Physics*, 7th ed. Springfield, Illinois: Charles C. Thomas, Publisher, 1985.

CHAPTER

6

Radiographic Tube and Radiation Production

CHAPTER OUTLINE

Introduction
Radiographic-Tube Construction
The Line Focus Principle
Tube Rating Charts
Tube Heat Capacity

OBJECTIVES

Upon completion of the chapter, the student will demonstrate knowledge, facts, and principles presented through oral and written evaluation and will meet the task objectives by demonstrating the specific behavior as identified in the terminal performance objectives of the procedures.

1. Describe and explain the function of the components of the radiographic tube as they relate to radiation production.
2. Describe radiographic tube heat production and show how to calculate its related heat capacity.
3. Explain the process by which radiation is produced from the conduction of electrons within the tube.
4. Explain radiographic tube stability related to heat production.

INTRODUCTION

In radiography, the X-ray machine is the primary instrument, and the radiographic tube is the most important part of this instrument. Yet, in day-to-day work, the radiographic tube is too often taken for granted—we tend to think the tube always functions properly until one day it no longer functions at all and has to be replaced. Generally, the tube seems to withstand a great deal of usage (and at times, abuse) but a knowledge of its operation can prevent many of the causes of tube failure.

RADIOGRAPHIC-TUBE CONSTRUCTION

The **X-ray tube** is a relatively simple instrument. Its structure consists of an outer metal housing, which serves as protection for the glass tube inserted within that housing, Figure 6-1. On one side of the tube is a source of electrons, the **cathode**. On the other side of the tube is the target for the electrons, the **anode**. Electrons are produced at the cathode in the **filament**.

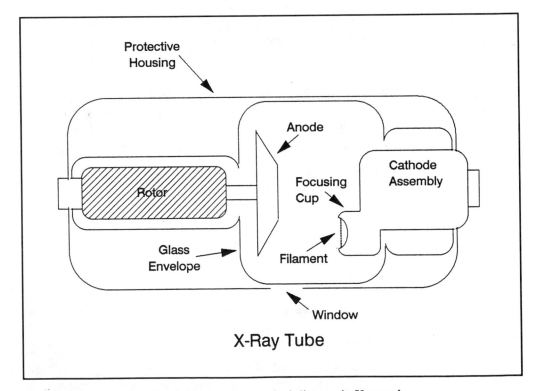

Figure 6-1. Cross-sectional diagram of a typical diagnostic X-ray tube

Most radiographic tubes have two filaments, a large and small one; such tubes are known as double focus tubes. The filaments are tungsten wire coils, which are set into **focusing cups**, Figure 6-2. The filament is heated by a high electrical **filament current**, which is measured in amperes. The current heats the tungsten (wire) and electrons are emitted from the filament in a process called **thermionic emission**. As the current is increased to the filament, the number of emitted electrons is increased. When the electrons are released, they collect in the space around the filament and remain there until electrical force is applied to move them. The force applied to move the electrons is measured in thousands of volts and is called kilovoltage (kV). The kilovoltage is applied through the potential difference across the tube, creating a net negative charge at the filament on the cathode side and a net positive charge at the target on the anode side. The kilovoltage force accelerates the electrons at a high velocity across the gap from the cathode to the

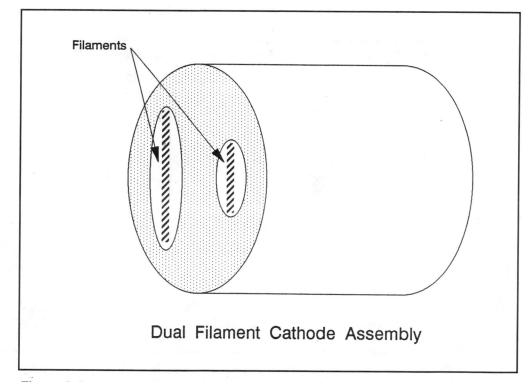

Figure 6-2. Dual filament focusing cup

anode, where they strike the part of the anode known as the **target**, Figure 6-3. The electron stream that flows between the cathode (negative) and anode (positive) makes up the **tube current**, measured in milliamperes (mA), and is sometimes called milliamperage.

The electron stream is focused on one part of the anode, called the target. The anode is made of tungsten and may be either a stationary wedge or a rotating disk. Tungsten is used because it has a very high melting point— 3410° C or 6170° F—and can therefore withstand much more heat than other metal materials. There is an enormous amount of heat created by the interaction of electrons in the anode, and tungsten is an excellent material for absorbing high degrees of heat. To help dissipate the large volume of heat, however, the anode may be made to rotate so that the heat is spread over the entire surface of the anode during exposure. Some tubes may be constructed with a rhenium-tungsten alloy anode that further reduces the heat load and subsequent thermal stress and may reduce the potential for surface roughening, cracking, or pitting.

Figure 6-3. Stationary anode *(left)* and rotating anode *(right)*

When the electrons are flowing at a high rate of speed and are stopped suddenly at the anode and interact with the anode, the production of radiant energy (X rays) occurs. Unfortunately, the kinetic energy is transformed mostly to heat (99 percent) and very little to useful X rays (1 percent), which is what is needed to produce the radiographic image. It is, however, the vast amount of heat production that may result in excessive tube heating.

As the electron stream strikes the anode surface, most of the X rays are projected perpendicular to the electron beam through the window opening (portal exit plane) in the tube housing (Figure 6-1). Tubes that are constructed with anodes that do not rotate have limited exposure capacity (i.e., dental units).

The radiographic tube has essentially been described, but further discussion of certain parts and their principal function is necessary. The tube components are enclosed in a glass envelope from which air has been removed. The tube must have as much gas or air removed as possible. Otherwise, the electrons would collide with gas molecules, thus reducing tube current. Also an evacuated tube has a longer life span and will not burn out as quickly.

A radiographic tube, like an electric light bulb, has a wire filament. A light bulb or an X-ray tube will burn out when the filament evaporates or becomes thinner. This occurs with age or usage when the tube is operated at maximum capacity. The radiographic machine itself is equipped with a double switch on the console (control panel). One switch, called the rotor, is used to heat the filament and to start the anode rotating to bring it up to the proper RPM (e.g., 3,000 or 10,000). The other switch actually makes the exposure. This also maintains control over the exposure. To reduce the amount of filament evaporation and extend the tube life, the rotor switch should only be used when the exposure is ready to be made. The radiographer should not hold the rotor switch on while instructing the patient. The small filament (corresponding to the small focal spot) may burn out faster than the larger one (corresponding to the large focal spot) depending on usage.

THE LINE FOCUS PRINCIPLE

The cathode (negative) side of the tube has been referred to several times. Electrons flow from negative (cathode) toward the positive (anode) side of the tube. The tungsten wire filament is mounted on the cathode in a cup-shaped depression, called the focusing cup, that serves to focus the electron beam on the anode target, Figure 6-4. The **line focus principle** is a result of the electron stream striking an angled target (i.e., ten degrees, twenty degrees). The part of the anode on which the electron beam impacts is called the **focal spot**. The effect is that of making the resulting X-ray beam smaller than the electron beam. Consequently, when an anode disk with less angle is used along with a small focal spot, the recorded image will have greater detail.

The electrons from the filament actually strike the anode in a rectangular shape, such as 1.0 mm × 3.0 mm, but effectively create an image on a film more square—1.0 mm × 1.0 mm. Thus, the radiographer must understand the difference between the **actual focal spot** and the **effective focal spot**. The size of the effective focal spot is based on 1) the angle of the tube and 2) the size of the filament.

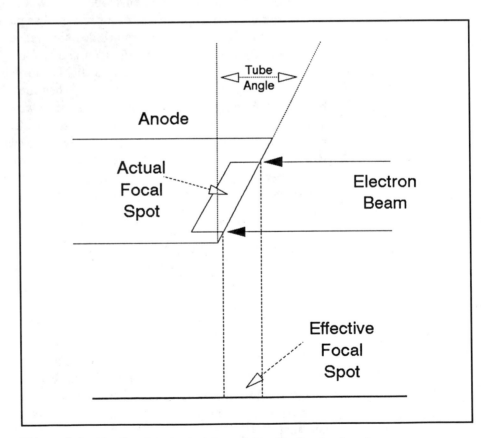

Figure 6-4. The line focus principle and the effective focal spot

TUBE RATING CHARTS

The purpose of a tube rating chart, Figure 6-5, is to extend the life of a tube and to assure that the tube can withstand the heat created by the workload. There are certain instantaneous ratings that are excessive and can seriously damage or cause a melting point on the tube anode surface. Such considerations include:

1. Never use high kVp on a cold target. The target must be warmed with several low exposures (low kVp, low mAs; i.e., 50 kVp 10 mA) before making a single high exposure. A tube target will become cold after about an hour of nonuse. Always warm the target when beginning the day's work or when the tube has cooled for a long period.
2. Never use an *excessive* single exposure, even on a warm anode.
3. The number of multiple exposures (e.g., twenty) that may be made at any given time must not exceed the tube's total heat capacity.
4. A radiographic tube that uses a fixed anode—one that does not rotate—is limited in its heat capacity and thus uses lower kVp and mA levels (i.e., dental unit).

Radiographers generally need only be concerned with warming a cold anode and not exceeding a single exposure rate on the anode. Remember, the rules for protecting and properly using a radiographic tube are easily followed through the manufacturer's recommendations included on rating charts that come with the tube purchase.

TUBE HEAT CAPACITY

Tube heat capacity has been referred to several times because the tube's problems are directly related to heat. Tube heat capacity is measured in heat units (HU). Heat units are simply a mathematical combination of exposure factors, kilovoltage (kVp), seconds (s), and milliamperage (mA) written in formula as kVp $\times$ s $\times$ mA. For detailed discussion about these exposure factors, refer to chapters 5 and 8. For now, let's say that the exposure factors 70 kVp $\times$ 1.0 seconds $\times$ 100 mA equal 7000 HU. Whether or not that number of HU would be more than the heat capacity of a given tube would depend on its total capacity and how much heat in HU had already been applied. Depending on the tube's intended workload, heat units vary from as little as 100,000 HU to 400,000 HU.

RATING CHARTS

Radiographic Rating Charts

Ratings for Three-Phase Full-Wave Rectification

Figure 6-5. Representative tube rating charts for a diagnostic X-ray tube

REVIEW QUESTIONS

1. The cathode beam of an X-ray tube is the
   a) primary X-ray beam
   b) focused electron beam within the tube
   c) current heating the filament
   d) secondary radiation

2. The target metal used in X-ray tubes should have the following two properties:
   a) high atomic number, high melting point
   b) low atomic number, low melting point
   c) low atomic number, high melting point
   d) high atomic number, low melting point

3. The process of boiling off of electrons from a hot, metallic filament is called
   a) Compton scatter
   b) pair production
   c) photoelectric effect
   d) thermionic emission

4. The positive terminal of an X-ray tube is the
   a) cathode
   b) anode
   c) focusing cup
   d) filament

5. The cloud of liberated electrons that remains in the vicinity of the hot filament is called
   a) tube current
   b) filament current
   c) positrons
   d) space charge

6. The negative terminal of an X-ray tube is the
   a) cathode
   b) anode
   c) target
   d) rotor

7. X rays are produced in the
   1) focal spot
   2) anode
   3) target
      a) 1 and 2
      b) 1 and 3
      c) 2 and 3
      d) 1, 2, and 3

8. The effective focal spot
   1) is smaller than the actual focal spot
   2) is on the anode

        3) determines the resolution
           a) 1 and 2
           b) 1 and 3
           c) 2 and 3
           d) 1, 2, and 3

9. A rotating anode
   1) dissipates heat
   2) has a larger target than a fixed anode
   3) is driven by an induction motor
      a) 1 and 2
      b) 1 and 3
      c) 2 and 3
      d) 1, 2, and 3

10. The tube housing
   1) helps contain scattered X rays
   2) is designed to aid in heat dissipation
   3) contains the glass envelope
      a) 1 and 2
      b) 1 and 3
      c) 2 and 3
      d) 1, 2, and 3

CHAPTER

7

Imaging Equipment

CHAPTER OUTLINE

Introduction
Radiographic Equipment
Primary and Secondary Circuits
  Primary Circuit
  Secondary Circuit
Types of Equipment
Accessory Items
  Calipers
  Cassettes

OBJECTIVES

Upon completion of the chapter, the student will demonstrate knowledge of the facts and principles presented through oral and written evaluation.

1. Explain permanently installed radiographic equipment and its maintenance.
2. Identify and discuss the various types and purposes of basic radiographic equipment.
3. Discuss the purposes, advantages, and disadvantages of routine and specific radiographic equipment.
4. Describe the purpose and disadvantages of mobile equipment and relate complexity of procedures.
5. Describe accessory equipment and the usage of different types.
6. Demonstrate competence in each task listed below. Refer to the appendix for the individual procedure/performance guides.

   TASKS (See Appendix):

   7-1 Cleaning radiographic facilities and equipment.
   7-2 Operating radiographic tables and consoles.

INTRODUCTION

This chapter deals with the electrical equipment needed to produce the radiographic image. It is important that prospective radiographers possess functional knowledge about the equipment they will use to practice their profession. Knowledge of the basis of the operation of radiographic units provides the radiographer with the background to use the imaging equipment most efficiently.

RADIOGRAPHIC EQUIPMENT

Radiographic equipment is the instrumentation needed for the performance of the tasks associated with radiographic procedures. Generally, we think of the permanently installed equipment—that which is used for either fluoroscopy or radiography, Figure 7-1. However, many items used as accessories in the production of radiographic images (e.g., grid cassettes, compression bands, etc.) are also considered radiographic equipment.

Figure 7-1. Permanently installed radiographic equipment *(Courtesy General Electric Medical Systems)*

The most important component of any radiographic unit is the tube. (The tube was discussed in detail in chapter 6.) The tube is a rotational or fixed part of a unit that also includes an electrical system and controls for circuits, generators, fuses, and switches. According to its purpose, a piece of equipment may be large, with many different components, or small, like a dental unit that hangs on the wall, Figure 7-2. All equipment must be handled with care and have regular maintenance, quality assurance, and testing to provide reliability.

Radiographic units may be divided into two basic parts: the primary circuit (also called the low-voltage circuit), and the secondary or high-voltage circuit.

Figure 7-2. Dental X-ray unit *(Courtesy General Electric Medical Systems)*

PRIMARY AND SECONDARY CIRCUITS

When a radiographic unit is installed, there must be a current source that comes from an outside source. The local utility company is responsible for the main supply of the incoming 110 or 220 volts of alternating current that will be used for any facility. Lines are brought in from outside and connected to a junction box inside, where the radiographic unit control console is connected.

To produce X rays, the line voltage must be controlled and changed to a direct current of many thousands of volts. This is done by the high-voltage transformer. A transformer is an electromagnetic device that will increase or decrease the voltage of alternating current. In an X-ray machine, the high-voltage transformer increases the low voltage of the primary circuit to the high voltage needed by the secondary circuit.

Primary Circuit

The primary circuit begins at the main power switch on the control console of the radiographic unit and leads to the primary coil of the high-tension transformer, Figure 7-3. Major components included in the primary section of the circuit are the autotransformer, kilovolt peak meter, voltage compensator, filament circuit, circuit breaker, and timers.

Autotransformer. This special type of transformer is used with the major and minor kVp selectors to provide a means to vary the voltage.

Kilovolt Peak Meter. This meter is connected to the autotransformer. Its function is to display the potential difference in kilovolts going to the high-voltage transformer.

Voltage Compensator. This component is connected across or in parallel with the primary circuit to the autotransformer. Its function is to increase or decrease the line voltage if there is a drop or surge in the line voltage.

Filament Circuit. The filament circuit is connected to the autotransformer. Its function is to supply current to the filament of the radiographic tube. The circuit supplies lower voltage and higher current by means of a step-down transformer, which is controlled by a rheostat or variable resistor.

Circuit Breaker. This is a protective device used to automatically terminate the current in the event that predetermined values are exceeded, i.e., excessive exposure or too much current from the line source. The breaker may be reset mechanically with a switch. If exposure factors cut off the breaker, then lower settings must be selected.

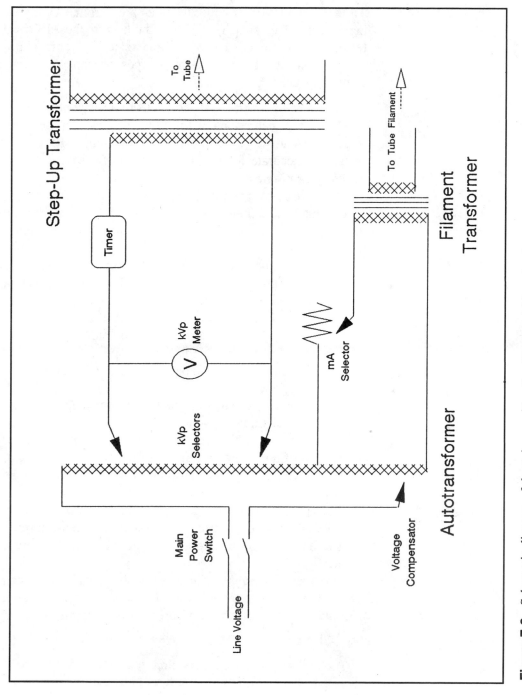

Figure 7-3. Schematic diagram of the primary side of an X-ray machine circuit

Timers.   Duration of exposure time is controlled by a switch in the timing circuit. The switch, which is built into the electrical circuit, will remain closed for the length of time selected by the radiographer at the control console or panel. Several types of exposure-timing devices are commonly used.

1. *Synchronous timers:* A synchronous timer is controlled and driven by an electrical synchronous motor. It is not generally used because it is not reliable and has limited exposure-time range. Exposure times are not usually accurate for shorter than 1/60 of a second.
2. *Electronic timers:*

    Impulse—A precise timing circuit that operates with an alternating current. The circuit is energized to variable time intervals, from milliseconds to seconds. It is accurate and may be used for rapid film production.

    mAs—A more specific electronic timer is used to control and terminate the time when the correct mAs is reached. This type of mAs timer is protection for tube current.
3. *Automatic timers:* A timing device that automatically terminates the exposure when the correct amount of radiation (density) has reached the film. The accuracy of this device depends on carefully positioning the anatomical part being radiographed correctly to the sensing element of the timing device.

    Automatic exposure-control devices are categorized as phototimer and ionization chamber.

    Phototimer utilizes a light-sensitive photomultiplier tube placed behind a fluorescent screen. The fluorescent screen, placed in front of or behind the film, produces light from radiation transmitted through the film. The light is picked up by the photomultiplier tube which terminates the exposure, after a predetermined charge that corresponds to the density of the film is reached. The amount of screen fluorescence (intensity) is directly proportional to the amount of radiation (intensity) that reaches the film.

    Ionization chamber utilizes a chamber located between the patient and the film. This chamber measures the amount of radiation reaching the film and shuts off the exposure at a predetermined setting.

Secondary Circuit

The high-voltage, secondary circuit begins with the secondary coil of the step-up transformer, Figure 7-4. It also includes the milliameter (mA), milli-

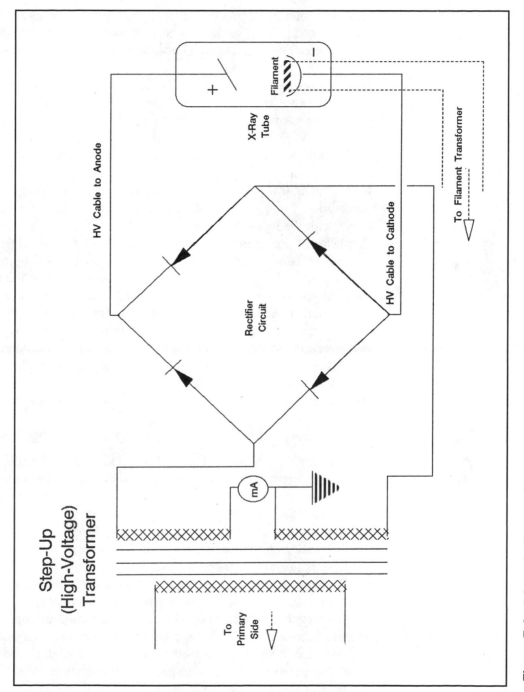

Figure 7-4. Schematic diagram of the secondary side of an X-ray machine circuit

ampere second meter (mAs), rectifiers, high-voltage cables and radiographic tube. All components of the secondary circuit are immersed in oil for purposes of electrical insulation and cooling in a separate section away from the radiographic unit console.

High-Voltage Transformer. The step-up, or high-voltage transformer consists of two iron coils wrapped with windings of electrical wire. The coil on the low-voltage side, carrying the current from the primary circuit, is called the primary coil. The coil on the high-voltage side carries the stepped-up, or increased voltage to the secondary circuit and is called the secondary coil.

Milliameter (mA). The mA meter is used to measure the current in milliamperes flowing through the radiographic tube. It is connected in series with the high-voltage circuit.

Rectifiers. Rectifiers are used to change alternating current to direct current, or current flowing in one direction, Figure 7-5. Alternating current is used in the primary circuit for two reasons: 1) it is the type of electricity supplied by the electrical utility, and 2) transformers will only work on alternating current. However, direct current is necessary to operate the radiographic tube so that electrons can be produced and kept flowing in one direction. Any reverse or change in current flow would cease electron production and could damage the tube. Rectification is controlled in modern equipment by devices called *diodes*. Modern radiographic equipment uses solid-state, silicone diode rectifiers to convert alternating current to direct current.

Two types of rectification are used in diagnostic radiology X-ray machines:

1. *Half-wave rectification*, Figure 7-5A. This type of rectification is used where current is directed by one or two diodes. Negative voltage is suppressed so that the flow of current is only utilized during the positive flow of alternating current. It is also called impulse current because one cycle of alternating current is applied.
2. *Full-wave rectification*, Figure 7-5B. This type of rectification is used in most radiographic units because it is the most efficient. It uses four diodes so that both the positive and negative impulses are used. There is a constant flow of positive current in one direction.

High-Voltage Cables. Two large cables are used to connect the radiographic tube to the high-voltage generator. One cable is attached to the cathode side of the tube; the other is connected to the anode side of the tube. The cables are designed to prevent any electrical hazard, such as arcing over of current flow from one terminal to the other.

Radiographic Tube. This component is the most important part of the radiographic unit. It is the component that creates the electrons that are used to produce the X rays that are the basis for radiographic images. Again, the tube is described in detail in chapter 6.

TYPES OF EQUIPMENT

Various types of units, either combined radiographic and fluoroscopic units (RF) or radiographic units only, may be found where radiographic images are produced. They may be installed for general or specific examination purposes, e.g., chest unit or head unit. In addition to installed units, there are portable units, used principally at the bedside. Important items of information to learn and remember about all radiographic units are:

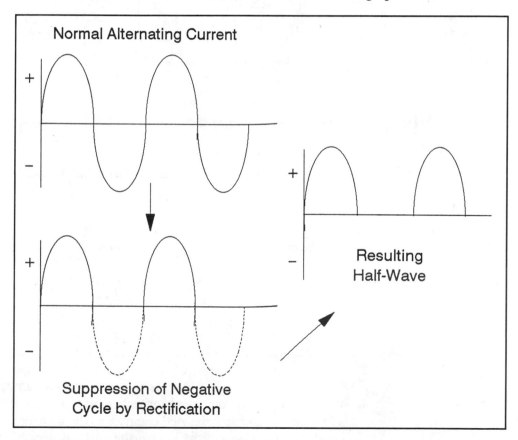

Figure 7-5A. Half-wave rectification of normal alternating current and the resulting waveform

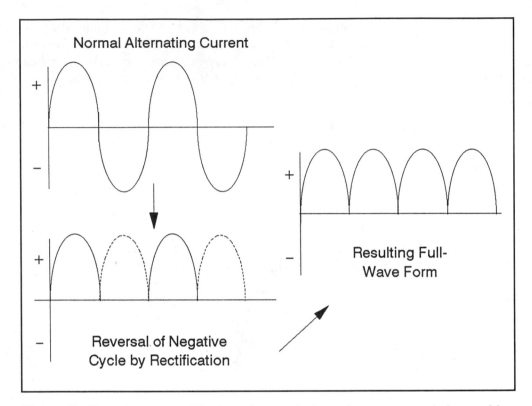

Figure 7-5B. Full-wave rectification of normal alternating current and the resulting waveform

1. *The electrical capacity of the unit in terms of milliamperage and kilovoltage.* Unless a radiographer is working with outdated equipment, a standard unit may have exposure ratings of from 100 to 1200 mA, kVp settings up to 150, and a dual focus tube (large and small focal spots). Other exposure factors include various time settings ranging from milliseconds to several whole seconds, i.e., 1/360–10 seconds, although radiographs are generally made at fractions of seconds.

2. *The limitation of any unit, especially portables.* In regard to portables, although the radiographer today is so concerned with limitation of exposure, the degree of equipment maneuverability is very important. That is, portable radiography may be complex when the patient's condition is unstable or body position must be maintained, as in orthopedic traction.

Extensive orthopedic traction for trauma patients usually requires an experienced radiographer's judgment for making films. Some specific units, such as head units, have limitations that restrict examining the patient who is either sitting or lying on a stretcher and cannot be moved. If the head unit is placed in a tight area or the radiographer does not understand its maneuverability, a head unit may become limited to use with the sitting position only.

3. *The purpose and combinations of exposure factors—the mA, time (s), and kVp selections.* The way in which all exposure factors affect the visible image must be clear to the radiographer. The function of all switches and meters on the control panel must be understood, Figure 7-6.

4. *The purpose and effectiveness of radiographic accessory items.* The way in which accessory items aid in the production or enhancement of the radiographic image is essential knowledge for the radiographer.

ACCESSORY ITEMS

Radiography uses numerous accessory items. Some may be unique to a particular radiographic procedure, such as those used in CT, MRI, or ultrasound. The most common items are cassettes, grid cassettes, calipers, film holders, film markers, film printers, compression bands, tape, and sponges. These items are generally found in any radiographic room. Although most are described and their uses explained in chapters 8 and 9, calipers and cassettes are discussed in this chapter.

Calipers

A caliper is a measuring device, used in radiography to measure the volume of tissue thickness of a body part. Tissue volume is a variable in exposure technique that must be accounted for in image production. It is a mistake to believe that one can simply and accurately visually judge tissue volume. Beyond a certain point, quality begins to suffer when one attempts to "guess" what every set of technical factors will be through visual estimation only. Moreover, it may often be useful for the radiographer measuring tissue volume with the caliper to be aware that tone and texture of tissues may be determined through touch. These discoveries, of course, cannot be made if one never measures tissue. Thus, we can see the deception of assuming exposure latitude. Exposure latitude allows for gradual margin of error

Figure 7-6. The control console of a diagnostic X-ray machine (*Courtesy General Electric Medical Systems*)

"of photographic effect" within certain kVp measurement ranges. It does not take into account conditions, such as ascites (abdominal fluid), where exposure must be manipulated to maintain equal photographic effect in density and contrast. The effect of tissue measurement may become less critical when some exposure factors are standardized and technique charts are developed on the basis of one-centimeter variations of tissue thickness. The radiographer may be able to visually evaluate tissue thickness by judging the distance between two lines that measure one centimeter.

To place the caliper properly, the (horizontal) sliding part of the device must be parallel to the base of the device and the vertical part must remain perpendicular to the base. The sliding part must not be pushed tightly against the tissue; it should be allowed to rest evenly along the part being measured. Measurement is always taken along the imaginary line where the central ray traverses the body part and at the same angle as the central ray. Extreme differences or variations in the part to be radiographed should be compensated by determining an average thickness within the total area of the part.

Automation of film processing and the use of faster imaging materials and exposure times only increase the essential need for the radiographer to determine exposure variables accurately. Tissue thickness and volume therefore must be taken into account no matter how exposure factors are determined.

Cassettes

A cassette is used to provide mechanical support and protection for the film and contains intensifying screens. Cassettes must be lightweight as well as lightproof, Figure 7-7.

Cassette fronts are made of material that offers almost no filtration to the passage of radiation. Because absorption of moisture may occur and cause expansion and contraction with temperature extremes, warping can result. Materials generally used in construction are: 1) a plastic that will absorb moisture but is radiolucent and 2) a metal alloy such as aluminum or magnesium.

Cassette backs are made of metal, aluminum, or steel. A thin sheet of foil may be attached to the inner side of the back of the cassette to prevent radiation from being scattered back through the cassette to fog film. In the case of photo-timed exposures, unnecessarily long exposures may result unless the phototube sensitivity is increased to sufficiently compensate for lead backing in the cassette.

Figure 7-7. Examples of X-ray film cassettes *(Courtesy General Electric Medical Systems)*

REVIEW QUESTIONS

1. Rectification is a process that changes
   a) direct current to alternating current
   b) alternating current to direct current
   c) high-voltage direct current to low-voltage direct current
   d) high-voltage alternating current to low-voltage alternating current

2. Self-rectification in an X-ray circuit leads to a voltage wave that is the same as
   a) full-wave
   b) half-wave
   c) direct current
   d) two of the above

3. Which of the following is found in the filament circuit?
   a) step-up transformer
   b) step-down transformer
   c) target
   d) exposure timer

4. Which of the following devices would be located between the secondary coil of the high-voltage transformer and the X-ray tube?
   a) rheostat (milliampere selector)
   b) rectifier
   c) autotransformer
   d) filament transformer

5. The function of the filament circuit is to
   a) supply low-voltage current to the anode
   b) supply high-voltage current to the filament
   c) supply low-voltage current to the filament
   d) supply high-voltage current to the autotransformer

6. Which of the following devices is found in the primary circuit?
   a) rectifier circuit
   b) X-ray tube
   c) autotransformer
   d) filament

7. Which type of X-ray timer terminates the exposure when a fluorescent screen produces light from the X rays?
   a) synchronous
   b) impulse
   c) mAs
   d) phototimer

8. Another name for a rectifier is
   a) autotransformer
   b) diode
   c) filament
   d) voltmeter

9. A device used to measure thickness of a body part is a
   a) caliper
   b) meter stick
   c) yard stick
   d) tape measure

10. Cassettes
    1) provide mechanical support for the film
    2) contain intensifying screens
    3) must be light proof
       a) 1 and 2
       b) 1 and 3
       c) 2 and 3
       d) 1, 2, and 3

CHAPTER

8

Fundamentals of Radiographic Exposure

CHAPTER OUTLINE

OBJECTIVES

Upon completion of the chapter, the student will demonstrate knowledge of the facts and principles presented through oral and written evaluation and will meet the task objectives by demonstrating the specific behavior as identified in the terminal performance objectives of the procedure.

1. Differentiate between the photographic and geometric properties related to the radiographic image.

2. Define and explain radiographic density as it relates to photographic properties of the radiographic image.
3. Define and explain radiographic contrast as it relates to photographic properties of the radiographic image.
4. Define other types of contrast: subject contrast, film contrast.
5. Define exposure latitude and kilovoltage ranges.
6. Explain what recorded detail means in the visible image.
7. Describe how mA, kVp, time, SID, and heel effect control and affect density and contrast in the radiographic image.
8. Explain the effect of motion on the formation of the radiographic image.
9. Explain the effect of magnification on the formation of the radiographic image.
10. Explain the effect of distortion on the formation of the radiographic image.
11. Given appropriate information, explain how to calculate exposure factors mA, time, kVp, and SID and their collective photographic effect.

INTRODUCTION

In this chapter the student will learn how to manipulate exposure factors according to their interactive effect on the radiographic image. Standardization of radiographic exposure factors, although theoretically based, must be understood in the application of day-to-day radiography. More importantly, the student must understand exposure latitude and how it provides a margin of error which varies depending on mathematical ranges of exposure factors (mA, time, kVp, SID). The quality of the visible radiographic image depends largely on the perception of the viewer. However, with a solid background in the knowledge of human anatomy and an understanding of the technical factors that create a radiographic image, the health professional is able to evaluate the image in discipline-specific terms.

IMAGE PRODUCTION

A radiograph is produced from X rays passing through a patient's body and interacting with the emulsion (surface) of a radiographic film. The finished radiograph is expected to provide a quality diagnostic image of the body part adjacent to the film. The image comprises the outlines and densities of the body part it represents (e.g., stomach, lungs). When processed with appropriate chemicals, the film emulsion yields a radiograph that, when placed on an illuminated light source (viewbox), provides visual information from which the physician can make a radiographic diagnosis.

A diagnostic quality radiograph should have adequate density (blackness), good contrast (range of gray shades), clear recorded detail (definition and resolution), and no visual distortion or magnification (size and shape) of the anatomy being examined. A physician interprets the anatomy in a radiograph based on visual properties. These properties can be categorized into two areas: density and contrast (categorized as photographic properties) and the recorded detail and absence of distortion and magnification (categorized as geometric properties). Table 8-1 summarizes the parameters for interpreting radiographs.

EXPOSURE FACTORS

Production of the visible radiographic image is controlled by the following exposure factors: milliamperage (mA), time, kilovoltage peak (kVp), and source-to-image distance (SID). However, other factors—heel effect, tube alignment to the film and body part, object-film distance, tissue thickness/pathology, screen selection, collimation and beam filters, fog, and film processing—also influence image production.

Exposure factors and other technical considerations will be discussed in the following paragraphs in relation to their effect on the image by photographic or geometric consequence. For the sake of simplicity, henceforth mA, time, kVp, and SID will be referred to as factors.

TABLE 8–1   IMAGE INTERPRETATION AREAS

PHOTOGRAPHIC PROPERTIES	GEOMETRIC PROPERTIES
Density	Recorded Detail
Contrast	Distortion
	Magnification

PHOTOGRAPHIC FACTORS

The two major photographic factors of the image are 1) *density* and 2) *contrast*.

Density

Density is seen as the overall blackness of the total image. Density is controlled by *milliamperage-seconds* (mAs)—it represents the quantity of radiation being produced for a certain length of time in an energized radiographic tube (as described in chapter 6). The mAs to be used during any given radiographic exposure, i.e., 100 mA, 200 mA, 300 mA, is set by the radiographer at the control console of the radiographic unit, Figure 8-1A & B. The density of the radiograph is directly proportional to the amount of mA used for exposure and length of time the exposure is delivered (referred to as mAs setting). A good principle to remember is that, proportionally, 200 mA will produce twice as much density on a film as will 100 mA. Higher mA selections will increase the production of electrons inside the tube (hence, quantity of radiation). Therefore, as more electrons are produced, more radiation reaches the film and more blackness or density will be seen on the film. Density is

Figure 8-1A. The control console is a modern, computerized panel. Only the exposure factors that have been selected are shown on the panel. Older machines may still show individual mA stations and the time (seconds) dial selector. *(Reprinted courtesy of Eastman Kodak Company)*

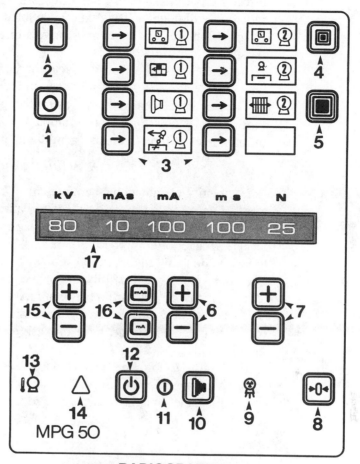

RADIOGRAPHY

1. Off key	9. X-RAY EXPOSURE signal lamp
2. On key	10. EXPOSE button
3. Auxiliary selection	11. EXPOSURE READY signal lamp
4. Small focal spot selection	12. PREP button
5. Large focal spot selection	13. HOUSING TEMPERATURE signal lamp
6. mA or mAs increment and decrement	14. PREP INHIBIT signal lamp
7. Exposure time increment and decrement	15. kV increment and decrement
8. Under exposure signal	16. 2- or 3-point mode selection
	17. Radiographic display

Figure 8-1B. Control console showing exposure factors selected for a specific exposure. Controls are defined in the key.

directly proportional to mA and time. If the mA is doubled, the quantity of radiation will double. If the time is doubled, the quantity of radiation will double. Both mA and time (mAs) have a direct effect on the degree of film darkening (density).

Time and Density.   Time is a factor of duration. It expresses the length of time that electrons (mA) are produced in the tube. As previously indicated, mA and time together are known as milliampere-seconds or mAs. Actually, time indicates how long a given amount of mA will last. In other words, milliamperes × time (seconds) = milliampere second (mAs). For example:

$$300 \text{ mA} \times 0.1 \text{ sec} = 30 \text{ mAs.}$$

The quantity of radiation, therefore, must be stated as mAs for four reasons: 1) mAs indicates quantity of radiation and how long the exposure lasted; 2) dosage is a product of mAs (e.g., a 300 mA selection and a time of one second would produce 300 mAs); 3) doubling the time has the same effect as doubling the mA (300 mA × 2 sec = 600 mAs; the quantity of radiation doubles and density or visible blackness in the recorded image doubles); 4) the relationship between mA × T should remain constant during repeated exposures as long as the radiation output is consistent and the generating equipment has been properly calibrated by a company service representative.

The fourth factor above is related to the *Reciprocity Law*. This law means that any combination of mA × T factors that are equivalent mAs should produce the same amount of density. See the following example for further elaboration.

mA	TIME(s)	CALCULATION	mAs
50	1/5 sec.	50 × 1/5 sec. =	10 mAs
100	1/10 sec.	100 × 1/10 sec. =	10 mAs
200	1/20 sec.	200 × 1/20 sec. =	10 mAs
300	1/30 sec.	300 × 1/30 sec. =	10 mAs

All of the above combinations should produce the same amount of density in the image (overall blackness). Thus, if a faster time is needed to avoid motion, mA and time may be changed according to the equation in the example.

Because time is a factor of duration, it is important to always identify the fastest exposure time compatible with other exposure factors (mA, kVp, SID) to avoid capturing any patient or organ motion in the recorded image.

Factors that control the mAs selection are: 1)the size of the focal spot to be used and 2)the amount of exposure time needed. Smaller focal-spot (filament) size in the tube results in sharper recorded detail of the anatomy seen in a radiographic image. For this reason, whenever practical, a smaller focal-spot size should be used. However, if the anatomy being radiographed is thick (large tissue volume, above 12 cm), a larger focal-spot size must be used due to the increased production of internal tube heat (see chapter 6). Thus, a disadvantage of the smaller focal-spot size is that it cannot tolerate the heat generated with the long or increased exposure time that may be required for thick body parts. The lower mA stations (i.e., 100 mA, 200 mA, and 300 mA) reflect a smaller focal spot. Larger focal-spot sizes are automatically switched on in the generator circuitry with larger mA selections (400 mA, 500 mA, 800 mA, and higher). The mA stations and their related focal-spot sizes vary with equipment and the particular heat unit capacity (HU) of the specific manufacturer's radiographic tube, Table 8-2.

Heat unit (HU) capacity has been discussed in chapter 6; however, subject matter is reiterated here for emphasis. The formula for determining HU capacity is:

$$mA \times T \times kVp$$

For example:

$$300 \text{ mA} \times 1 \text{ sec} \times 80 \text{ kVp} = 24000 \text{ HU}$$

If the total tube capacity is 300,000 HU, then the exposure cited in the example would use only a small portion (0.08%) of the total capacity. The tube therefore could still withstand much more heat, which would allow several more exposures within the same range.

Other factors that interact to change the direct effect of density are *kVp*, *SID*, *heel effect*, *film processing*, and *fog*.

Quantity of radiation for technique charts may be determined by trial and error using various combinations of mA × T on a phantom or device that represents the equivalency of human body structure. *Never use real human subjects* to establish technique factors. Once the average adult quantity of radiation has been established for a given part of the body, e.g., head or chest, it is seldom necessary to adjust the mA. Only the time factor and sometimes the kilovoltage will need to be adjusted for various thickness ranges of anatomical structures. Table 8-3 shows examples of time variations.

TABLE 8–2   ADVANTAGES/DISADVANTAGES OF SMALL AND LARGE FOCAL SPOTS

FOCAL-SPOT SIZE (FSS)	ADVANTAGES	DISADVANTAGES
Smaller Focal Spot (100, 200, 300 mA stations)	Use results in greater recorded detail of image.	Longer (slower) exposure time may result in patient motion. Focal spot cannot tolerate heat generated by a long exposure time.
Larger Focal Spot (400, 500, 800 mA stations)	Shorter (faster) exposure time minimizes risk of patient motion. Focal spot can tolerate increased heat generated by longer exposure times.	Use results in loss of recorded detail of image.

TABLE 8–3   EXAMPLES OF TIME VARIATIONS FOR AVERAGE ADULT CHEST

CHEST	mA	cm MEASUREMENT	T	mAs
	300	Small 15–18	1/30	10
	300	Medium 19–22	1/15	20
	300	Large 25–32	1/10	30

Note: The chart shows how the time can be adjusted to accommodate various chest-size ranges without changing the mA. However, these calculations may not be appropriate for a given radiographic unit.

kVp and Density. kVp controls contrast. It does, however, affect density in two ways. As kVp is increased, the stream of electrons in the tube moves more efficiently across the tube and results in increased part penetration (discussed later with kVp). A second effect is that as kVp is increased, more radiation energy is produced, resulting in more scattered radiation, which increases density to the film (recorded image). This can be controlled by use of a grid (discussed under Accessories).

Distance and Density. Distance, or source-to-image distance (SID), has a significant influence on density. The effect of distance on density (SID) obeys the *inverse square law*, Figure 8-2. Understanding the concept

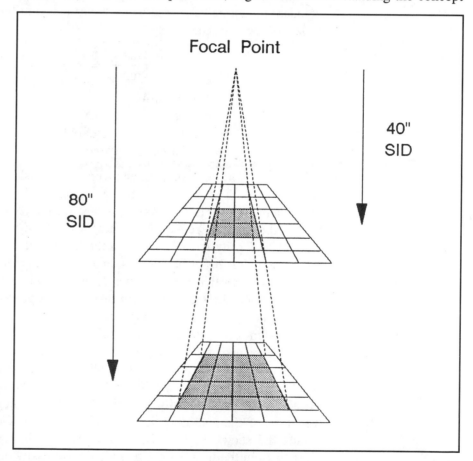

Figure 8-2. At forty inches, a four-square area represents the SID spread. At eighty inches, twice the distance, a sixteen-square area represents the SID and shows increased spread for the same quantity of radiation.

of the inverse square law is necessary because it relates to density, radiation intensity, and radiation dosage. The inverse square law states: *The intensity of radiation is inversely proportional to the square of the distance.* That is, if forty inches SID is increased to eighty inches SID, the radiation beam spreads over an area four times greater and its intensity diminishes by a factor of four. A change in distance (SID) requires a new mAs value in order to obtain the same amount of density on the radiograph. If the SID is changed to eighty inches from forty inches, a new mAs value is needed to prevent film density from being very light or underexposed. In order to obtain the same amount of density at eighty inches, more initial radiation exposure is required as based on the inverse square law. The following formula may be applied:

$$\frac{mAs_1}{mAs_2} = \frac{d_1^2}{d_2^2}$$

Where: mAs_1 = original mAs
        mAs_2 = new mAs
        d_1^2 = original distance squared
        d_2^2 = new distance squared

The above formula expresses an inverse relationship between SID changes and new mAs. Therefore, making any change in the SID requires a change in milliamperage or time (mAs). A change from forty inches to eighty inches SID is the same as reducing the radiation intensity four times. Thus, the amount of density reduction seen in the image occurs because the intensity of the radiation beam has been attenuated or thinned out over four times more area when twice the distance is used, Table 8-4.

Simply put, the radiation beam diverges and proceeds in a straight path (lines). The area covered becomes increasingly larger with lessened intensity as the beam of radiation travels a greater distance from the source. To produce a given density at a different distance, it is necessary to vary the exposure inversely with the square of the distance. The exposure area in Figure 8-2 has increased four times from 40 inches to 80 inches.

Heel Effect and Density. Heel effect is a phenomenon related to the structure of the radiographic tube, i.e., the tube's target (anode) angle. Figure 8-3 shows the long axis of the tube and how the radiation beam is emitted from the focal spot. The radiation intensity diminishes along a line parallel with the long axis of the tube, i.e., the heel effect. As shown in Figure 8-3A, the intensity of the exposure increases toward the cathode

TABLE 8-4 EXAMPLES BASED ON USE OF THE INVERSE SQUARE LAW							
A INCREASE IN SID (DOUBLED)*				B DECREASE IN SID (HALVED)**			
SID	mAs	SID	mAs	SID	mAs	SID	mAs
40	30	80	120	40	30	20	7.5

$$\frac{*30 \text{ mAs}}{x} = \frac{40^2 \text{ SID}}{80^2}$$

$$\frac{30 \text{ mAs}}{x} = \frac{1600 \text{ SID}}{6400}$$

$$1600x = 192000$$

$$x = 120 \text{ new mAs}$$

$$\frac{**30 \text{ mAs}}{x} = \frac{40^2 \text{ SID}}{20^2}$$

$$\frac{30 \text{ mAs}}{x} = \frac{1600 \text{ SID}}{400}$$

$$1600x = 12000$$

$$x = 7.5 \text{ new mAs}$$

Note: Using the inverse square law formula, Column A shows the increased mAs that would be necessary if the SID was doubled from 40 to 80 as seen in Figure 8-2. Column B shows the decreased mAs that would be necessary if the SID was reduced (halved) from 40 to 20.

(filament) side of the tube while it decreases toward the anode (target) side of the tube as a result of the target angle. This creates more radiation to be emitted at the cathode side of the tube. The effect is more pronounced in tubes with steeper target angles (10 degrees) than in tubes with greater target angles (20 degrees), Figure 8-3B. The heel effect should be utilized to equalize the exposure distribution over various-thickness tissue densities.

The rule should be to align the long axis of the tube parallel with the longer or broader portion of the anatomical structure being examined so that the cathode side of the tube is directed over the thicker part of the structure. One example for proper tube alignment is radiographic examination of the femur. The cathode side of the tube should be directed toward the hip region and the anode side over the knee region so that the more intense radiation

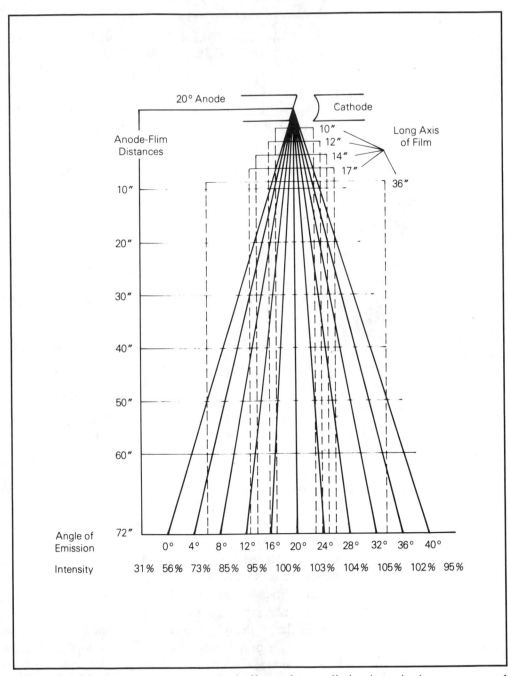

Figure 8-3A. Representation of the heel effect, where radiation intensity increases toward the cathode end of the tube

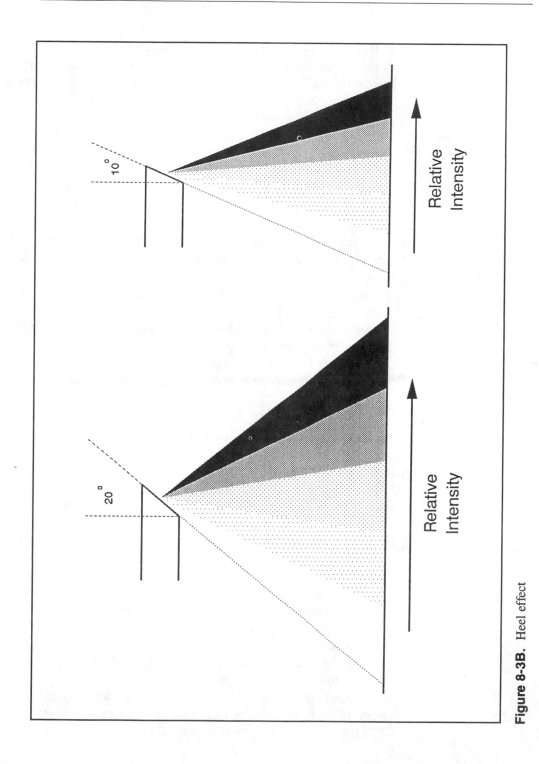

10°

20°

Relative
Intensity

Relative
Intensity

Figure 8-3B. Heel effect

will pass through the adjacent thicker upper femoral area. Another example is the examination of the lower leg. The cathode side should be directed toward the knee thickness or proximal leg to balance radiation distribution. A final example is a lateral lumbar spine. The cathode side of the tube should be directed over the upper pelvic region.

Film Fog and Density.   Density may also be affected by film fog, which is unwanted density that makes it difficult to visualize structures on the radiograph. Film fog may be caused by age (old film), light (result is total blackening of film emulsion), scattered radiation exposure, or improper film development. In order to prevent or reduce film fog, the darkroom must be lightproof. The darkroom safelight should be well-positioned and maintained. Film must be used according to its expiration date. Radiographic film must be processed properly, and unused film should be stored in a lead-lined room or container. Any change in processing time or temperature will quickly affect density in a radiograph. Chapter 9 discusses in more detail why time and temperature must remain constant.

Artifacts are foreign or unwanted marks that show up on a radiograph because of improper film handling, improper processing, or faulty equipment. Artifacts can result in a change (either an increase or a decrease) in film density, usually in a particular area of the image.

Contrast

Contrast is the second major photographic factor. There are three types of contrast: radiographic, subject, and film. Each will be discussed as their role in a diagnostic quality radiograph.

Radiographic contrast results from the distribution of black metallic silver in the film emulsion and is directly controlled by the penetrating effects of kilovoltage. Radiographic contrast is visualized in the image as gray tones or degrees of gray that reveal the differences between body organs or tissues. Contrast enhances information. If no contrast can be seen between organs, then very little information may be visible in the radiographic image. An excellent example of this phenomena in human anatomy is an obese abdomen where the internal organs appear as equal in tissue thickness and therefore density because of fat content. It is like looking for a white goose in a snow storm. Contrast is controlled by the kilovoltage or, more technically, the quality of energy or wavelength (short or long). You may want to refer to the chapter on physics, chapter 5.

A variety of long and short wavelengths (low and high energies) will demonstrate a range of shades from black to gray to white (gray tones) density differences. The differences are easily seen in the structures visible in the radiographic image. In the blacker portion of a radiograph, the visible structures will have absorbed *less* radiation, and the whiter portion of the visible structures will have absorbed *more* radiation. This means that the whiter structures have greater tissue density.

Radiographic contrast is generally referred to as the overall contrast seen in the image. It includes long-scale (more gray tones) contrast and short-scale (more black and white tones) contrast. Radiation of higher energy (shorter wavelength), 70 kVp or more, will produce long-scale contrast with many gray tones, Figure 8-4A. Additionally, tissues having little difference in thickness or density will appear as images with flat gray tones. If there are large differences in the thickness of body structures, e.g., bone vs. soft tissue, or if 70 kilovoltage and lower is used, short-scale contrast with more pronounced black and white tones will be produced, Figure 8-4B. Much of

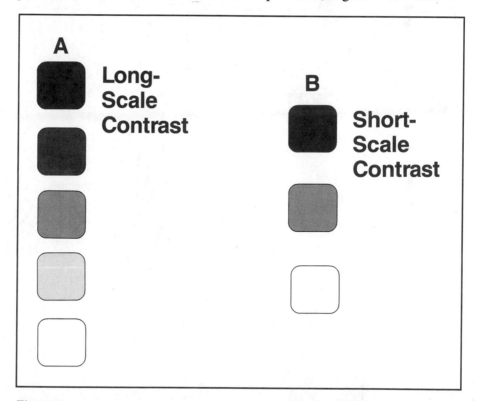

Figure 8-4. A) In long-scale contrast, several degrees of gray to black tones will be produced in the image with higher kVp ranges, i.e., above 70 kVp; B) In short-scale contrast, the range of gray tones is more abrupt from white to black. Fewer gray tones will be seen in the image. Short-scale contrast is produced at lower kVp ranges, i.e., below 70 kVp.

the radiographic image contrast is influenced by *subject contrast* and *film contrast*.

Subject contrast depends on how much the radiation beam is attenuated or thins out as it enters, passes through, and exits the various structures within the body. This is what is known as an *aerial image*, which is created by the absorption of radiation in various percentages by different tissue thicknesses, Figure 8-5. Bone will absorb more radiation than soft tissue, but this may vary greatly depending on tissue density, age, disease, or other conditions where structure may change or be complex.

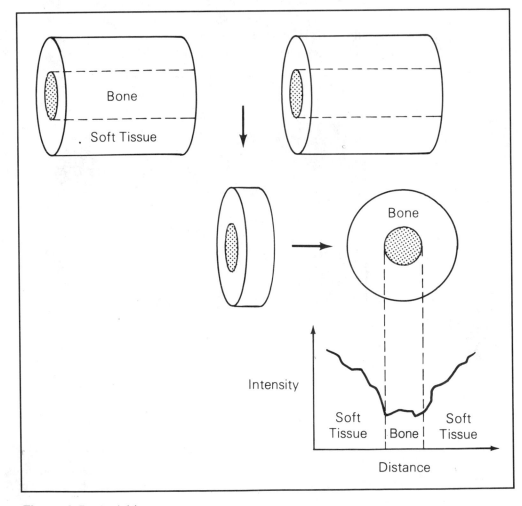

Figure 8-5. Aerial image

Film contrast is inherent in the type of filming system being used, including 1) the type of film (low-contrast or high-contrast), 2) the processing conditions (the time-temperature method of developing films should be adhered to for visualization of optimal contrast—see chapter 9), and 3) the use of screens versus no screens. That is, because intensifying screens convert radiant energy to visible light, contrast is increased with screens; whereas without screens (direct exposure), contrast is affected mostly by the natural difference in tissue thickness.

As previously stated, contrast enhances information by making the detail of structures appropriately visible in the image. Without appropriate levels of subject contrast being visualized in the radiographic image, it would be difficult to differentiate human structures and diseases with discernible accuracy.

It was stated earlier, under the discussion on mAs, that the overall amount of density or blackness seen in the radiographic image is controlled by the quantity of mAs used and that the degree of density is proportionate to the mAs (double the mAs, double the density). By comparison, contrast is controlled by kVp and has an approximate effect on the image according to the 15 percent rule. This rule means that if you are using 80 kVp in your technique factors (i.e., 300 mA, .30 seconds, 80 kVp) and you add 15 percent (12 kVp) more to the original 80, kVp is increased to 92. Such a change would double the kVp penetration effectiveness, but contrast would visibly decrease.

Increasing the kVp by 15 percent has an effect equivalent to increasing or decreasing the mAs by one half. It should be noted that although kVp and mAs have an interactive effect in increasing or decreasing contrast and density respectively, they may not be interchanged to compensate for the lack of one or the other. As further explanation, note that if structures are underpenetrated due to a lack of kVp, no amount of mAs increase will improve the penetration; added mAs will only add density. Penetration of structure can best be achieved by using the appropriate amount of kVp. Conversely, if an image is underexposed and lacks density, mAs must be added; kVp would add only scattered radiation and thus cause the image to look gray and flat without clarity.

In summary, the two factors of mAs (density) and kVp (contrast) must be used so that the interactive effects are complementary to each other and not compensatory for the lack of one or the other.

Milliamperage-Seconds (mAs) and Contrast. Milliamperage-seconds (mAs) fundamentally controls the quantity of radiation; kVp fundamentally controls contrast. The two factors must not be interchanged. Too much mAs will result in increased density or blackness with an accompanying loss of visible radiographic contrast. It is equally important to note that increasing mAs generally will not improve structure penetration which is also controlled by kVp.

Distance and Contrast (kVp).   The intensity of primary and secondary radiation changes inversely proportional to the square of the distance. Any change in distance will result in a proportionate change in the amount of scattered radiation. Thus, image contrast will not be affected. The degree of density in nearby structures may be lighter or darker, but the level of contrast will be fundamentally unchanged. Additionally, the degree of structure penetration will not, for all practical purposes, be affected. Levels of kVp penetration are equally effective at any distance (e.g., 70 kVp, 80 kVp).

Other Factors and Density and Contrast.   Other factors that influence both density and contrast are beam restriction, beam filtration, and compression of tissue. Although these areas are discussed later in the chapter, they are mentioned here to facilitate easy reference.

Beam restriction or *limitation* reduces the amount of scattered radiation interacting with the body and thereby prevents excessive scatter from fogging the film with increased density and decreased contrast of the visible image.

Beam filtration (filters) is added to the radiation beam to eliminate non-useful soft, low-energy (long wavelengths) radiation. This filtration results in hardening of the beam by allowing mostly higher energy (shorter wavelengths) to pass through unchanged. Contrast may be improved then with a decreased amount of lower-energy wavelengths.

Compression of tissue has the effect of reducing tissue thickness. In the area where tissue is compressed, therefore, contrast may be visibly reduced due to increased penetration by kVp. Density will be increased in the same area due to less absorption of radiation in an area of compression.

GEOMETRIC FACTORS

Density and contrast are photographic factors that refer to the properties of the visible radiographic image. Geometric factors deal with the recorded detail of the image and how accurately the true edges of the anatomy may be seen. *Recorded detail*, *distortion*, and *magnification* are the geometric factors of interest.

Recorded Detail

Recorded detail is the degree of information or definition that may be seen in the anatomy or the resolution or sharpness of lines that separates one structure from another. Although motion is rarely seen in a radiographic image because of very rapid exposure-time settings on today's equipment, motion, nevertheless, completely destroys information by blurring the image. It really does not require a great deal of experience or knowledge to recognize blurring in a radiographic image. It may be compared to the blurring seen in an ordinary photograph when the subject has moved. The fastest possible exposure time therefore is the best recourse against motion and should always be used in accordance with all other factors when making any radiographic exposure.

Focal-spot size (FSS), source-to-image-distance (SID), object-film distance (OFD), and intensifying screens are factors that influence the geometry of the image, and each must be designed to reduce or minimize the geometric blur. "Geometric blur," or penumbra, Figure 8-6, is the term used to describe the gradient unsharpness or edge enhancement of an image.

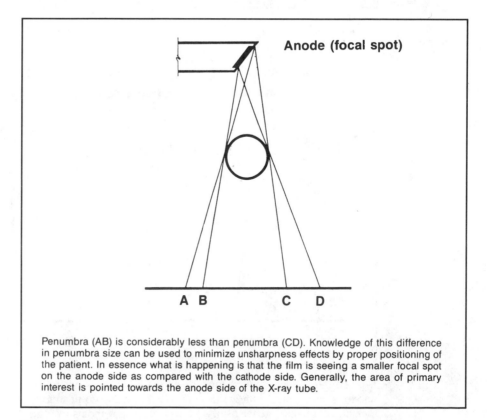

Penumbra (AB) is considerably less than penumbra (CD). Knowledge of this difference in penumbra size can be used to minimize unsharpness effects by proper positioning of the patient. In essence what is happening is that the film is seeing a smaller focal spot on the anode side as compared with the cathode side. Generally, the area of primary interest is pointed towards the anode side of the X-ray tube.

Figure 8-6. Focal spot and its relationship to subject placement *(Reprinted courtesy of Eastman Kodak Company)*

Focal-Spot Size. The effective focal-spot size was discussed in chapter 6. The relationship of the focal spot to geometric blur is that it is the single most important factor in recording the detail of the anatomy in the radiographic image. The smaller focal spot (produced by the smaller filament) in a dual focus tube will produce more recorded detail than the larger focal spot (filament), Figure 8-7. The rule to follow in utilizing focal-spot size is to use the smaller one whenever the exposure factors (mA, T, kVp, and SID) are set low enough to allow its use.

Source-to-Image Distance. SID, for all practical purposes, has no effect on the penetrating power of the kVp. Changes in the SID will not affect contrast as long as the kVp remains unchanged. The rule concerning the relationship between SID and recorded detail is that a greater (increased)

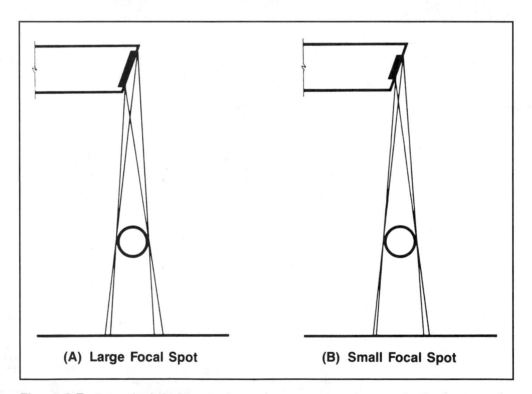

(A) Large Focal Spot   **(B) Small Focal Spot**

Figure 8-7. Penumbral shadow or edge unsharpness occurs because the focal spot on the anode is not a point source. It is comprised of many point sources, each of which projects its own object image onto the film. A) Large focal spot and its resulting penumbra; B) Small focal spot and a reduced amount of penumbra. *(Reprinted courtesy of Eastman Kodak Company)*

SID will reduce geometric blur and thus improve recorded detail. (See the penumbra reduction in Figure 8-8.) Most radiographic images are produced at a standardized forty-inch SID.

Object-Film Distance (OFD). OFD may also be referred to as object-image distance (OID). Either term refers to the practice/rule of placing the anatomy (object) as close to the film (in the cassette holder) as possible. This is a cardinal rule to observe in radiography because magnification occurs when the part is not close to the film. The result is an overall enlarged and fuzzy image. Although we recognize that placing the anatomy adjacent to the film surface is not always possible, minimizing the gap is

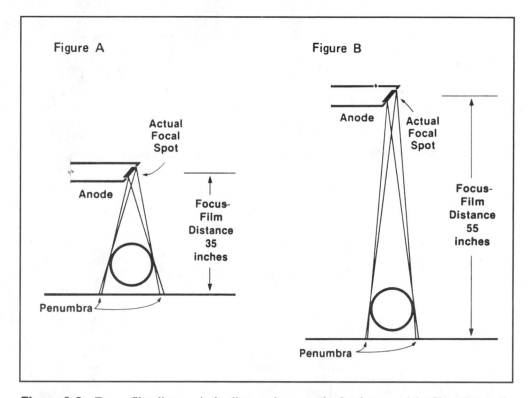

Figure 8-8. Focus-film distance is the distance between the focal spot and the film. Generally speaking, focus-film distance directly affects the degree of penumbral shadow and geometric unsharpness. Note that in the illustrations below, figure A had a 35-inch focus-film distance and has a greater degree of penumbral shadow than figure B which has a 55-inch focus-film distance. The radiographic illustrations provided graphically illustrate the difference in penumbral shadow as one goes from a short focus-film distance to a long focus-film distance. *(Reprinted courtesy of Eastman Kodak Company)*

important to reducing geometric blur, Figure 8-9. The rule should be to always place the part (object) adjacent to or as close as possible to the cassette surface.

Intensifying Screens. Intensifying screens affect recorded detail according to the size of the phosphor crystal (see chapter 9). Smaller crystal size will create less blurring of the image because there is less diffusion of light created by the smaller crystal, Figure 8-10. Screens are discussed in greater detail under Accessories.

Screen-Film Contact. The loss of screen film contact is infrequent with automatic systems where no one ever touches or opens cassettes.

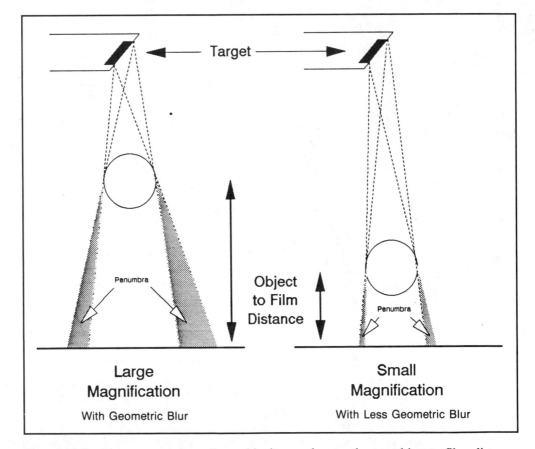

Figure 8-9. Improvement in radiographic image due to shorter object-to-film distance *(Reprinted courtesy of Eastman Kodak Company)*

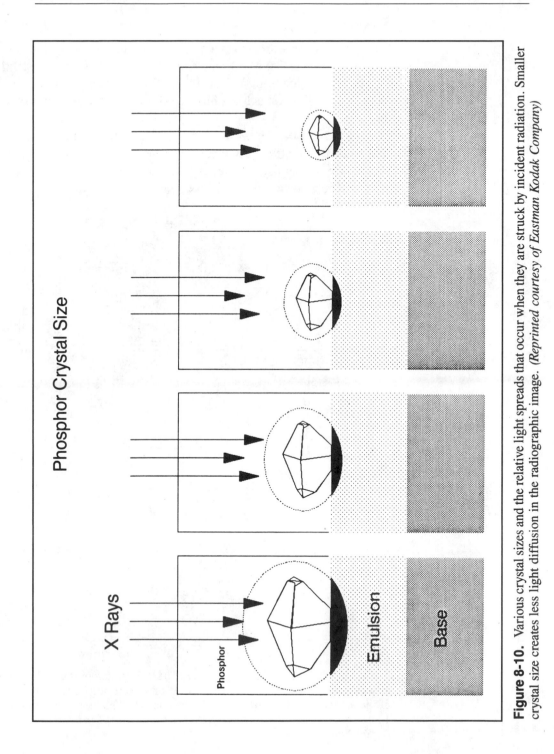

Figure 8-10. Various crystal sizes and the relative light spreads that occur when they are struck by incident radiation. Smaller crystal size creates less light diffusion in the radiographic image. *(Reprinted courtesy of Eastman Kodak Company)*

Generally, screen-film contact is lost only in cassettes that are larger in size (14 × 17 in/35 × 43 cm) and when cassettes are constantly opened for loading, unloading, and cleaning. What visually appears with incomplete screen-film contact is a blurring of the image, usually in the center of the film.

Film Resolution.   Film resolution is the ability of the crystals within the film emulsion to efficiently record information. This ability is dependent on crystal size. Generally, smaller crystal size will be able to resolve and record more image information with less geometric blur than larger crystal size.

Figure 8-11.   Poor screen film contact. These films demonstrate blurring around the areas where the coins have been placed. Poor screen film contact appears in the area of the screens where there may be poor contact. This is more common with large 14×17 size screens than with any other size screens. *(Reprinted courtesy of Eastman Kodak Company)*

Distortion and Magnification

Distortion of the radiographic image refers to changes in size or shape of the anatomic part (as seen in real life and projected on the radiograph). Magnification, foreshortening, and elongation of the actual image size or shape are forms of distortion. A number of factors—object-to-film distance (OFD), distance (SID), motion, focal-spot size (FSS), and tube-to-part alignment—influence geometric factors, Figure 8-11, although they do not control them.

Motion. Motion is a major factor in reducing image clarity and increasing distortion. A radiograph containing motion is referred to as a "blurred image." The blurred or fuzzy edges result in increased penumbra. Using as fast an exposure time as possible and patient immobilization devices are the best methods to reduce image distortion caused by motion.

Tube-Part Alignment. Improper alignment of the tube or central ray to the body part or the film results in distortion. This distortion may cause the image to appear longer or shorter than its actual length. The physical shape of the anatomic part can also influence the amount of distortion. Whenever possible, to avoid shape distortion, the radiographic tube (central ray) should be perpendicular to the long axis of the part, Figure 8-13.

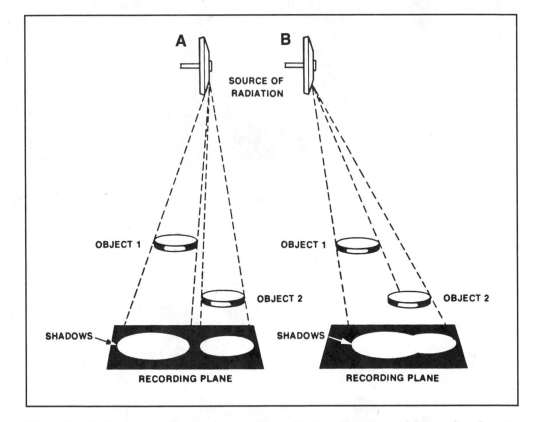

Figure 8-12. Some magnification in the radiographic image may be useful (e.g., for a finger). Distortion, however, is rarely helpful. A) No distortion in the circular objects on the recording plane (film); B) With a change in the direction (angle) of the radiation, the circular objects elongate and overlap—they appear as one object. The radiation must pass through the object perpendicularly as the object is placed parallel to the recording plane.

IMAGE-PRODUCTION ACCESSORIES

There are several accessory items that are very important to image production. These accessory items are generally standardized and few changes need ever be made regarding their use and application. It is important however to understand the purpose of and effect of these items on the image. These accessory items are: *intensifying screens*, *grids*, *beam restrictors*, *filtration*, and *processing*.

Intensifying Screens

Intensifying screens have phosphors that intensify the action of radiation. Although screens are addressed in chapter 9, some review is appropriate

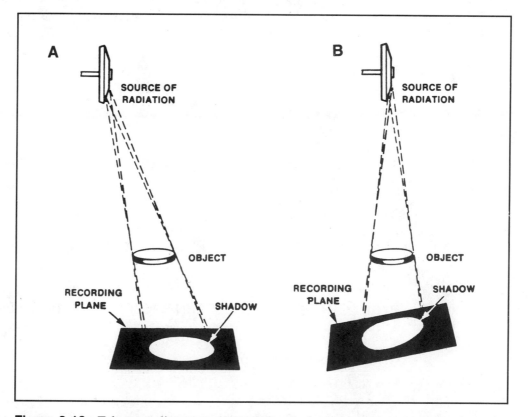

Figure 8-13. Tube-part alignment. A) Even though the source is not vertically above the circular object, it casts a circular shadow, provided the object and the recording plane are parallel; B) Distortion results when object and image-receptor plane are not parallel.

here to help understand the effect of exposure with screens. Two important elements of screens are: 1) the size of the crystal and 2) thickness of the layer of the phosphor. The effect that screens have on density is related to both the crystal size and thickness of the emulsion, which determines the screen speed (response time) or amount of light produced (intensification). There are several categories of screens: detail or slow-speed screens, general purpose or medium-speed screens, and fast or high-speed screens. For convenience and ease of recognition, screen speeds have been given specific numbers by manufacturers. Some related information appears in Table 8-5.

Screen-speed factor or intensification of screens is determined as a ratio of the amount of exposure necessary without screens to the amount necessary with screens:

$$\text{Intensification factor} \atop \text{(speed factor)} = \frac{\text{exposure without screens}}{\text{exposure with screens}}$$

TABLE 8–5 RELATIVE SCREEN SPEED FOR GREEN-SENSITIVE (RARE-EARTH) AND BLUE-SENSITIVE SCREENS

GREEN-LIGHT-EMISSION SCREEN SPEED	RELATIVE SPEED
Detail (slow)	80–100
General purpose (medium)	250–300
Fast (high)	400–800
Ultrahigh	1200
BLUE-LIGHT-EMISSION SCREEN SPEED	**RELATIVE SPEED**
Detail (slow)	20–30
General purpose (medium)	100–200
Fast (high)	250

Note: This table lists only a few generalized screen speeds. Detailed charts showing related film types may be obtained from the appropriate screen manufacturer.

Because we are concerned with the amount of density produced in the combination of screens and film, it is more effective and efficient to think in terms of speed. That is, if one is in the process of changing screens, it is necessary to know what change in exposure factors, if any, will be required. For example, a speed factor of 100 would require 50 percent more exposure than a speed factor of 200 (see Table 8-5).

Screen speed affects density by the required exposure necessary to produce a given amount of blackness in the radiographic image. Again, using the above factors, if a general purpose screen with a rating of 200 is used and it is then decided that a detail screen with a rating of 100 is needed, an increase of 50 percent more exposure will be needed to maintain the same density with the slower detail screen. For practical purposes, however, the daily use of screens is standardized, so that exposure factors are determined according to the way in which radiographic procedures are conducted on a routine basis. Procedures may vary from extremities, chest, abdomen, pelvis, spine, and skull examinations in large radiography departments to extremities, chest, abdomen, and pelvis in smaller departments or a doctor's office.

Grids

Grids are precision instruments designed for the single purpose of absorbing scattered radiation, although some primary radiation is absorbed as well. A grid is designed to be used where density of the image is affected by the amount of scattered radiation reaching the film. This is because a greater exposure is needed for producing images of structures that measure above 12 cm in thickness where more than 70 kVp is required. When kVp settings are increased, more scattered radiation is created. Basically, changing from no grid to the use of a grid requires four times more exposure because of scattered and primary beam absorption by lead strips in the grid, Figure 8-14. The grid works in this way: when a grid is added, it is placed under the table, between the patient and the film. The lead strips in the grid absorb divergent radiation beams scattered away from the direction of the more perpendicular primary beam. The gaps between the lead strips allow the primary beam to reach and interact with the film emulsion whereas the scattered radiation is absorbed by the lead strips. The amount of scattered radiation that is absorbed by the grid is related to *grid ratio*. Grid ratio is defined as the ratio of the height of the lead strips to the distance between the lead strips, as seen in the following diagram, Figure 8-15.

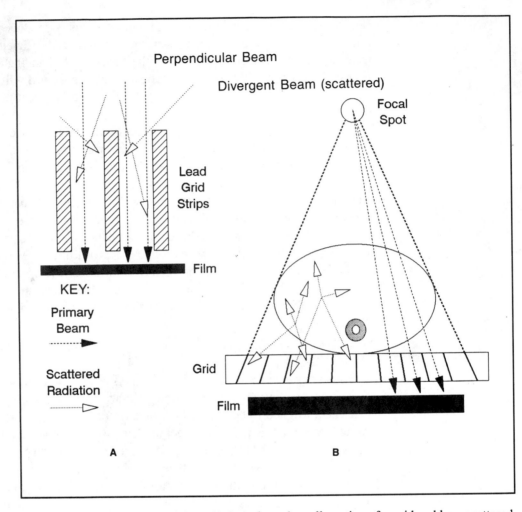

Figure 8-14. Grid cross section. A) An enlarged small portion of a grid and how scattered radiation is absorbed by the lead strips. It also shows how perpendicular radiation from the primary beam passes between the lead strips to reach the film emulsion. B) The radiation of the radiation beam, the part being examined, the grid, and the image-recording receptor.

As seen in the diagram, the effect of the grid lines, or its efficiency (cleanup ability) depends on the height of the lead strips and the distance between the strips (wide or narrow). The less the distance between them and greater the height, as in the 16:1 ratio, the more efficient the grid will be in pickup or removal of scattered radiation.

Figure 8-15. Effect of grid ratio on scatter angle

Approximately four times more mAs must be added when a grid is used than when a grid is not used because of absorption by the lead strips. Otherwise, there would be a loss of density that would cause the radiographic image to appear greatly underexposed. For example, if 5 mAs is used without a grid, 20 mAs must be used with a grid. (See grid conversion chart, Table 8-6.)

Beam Restriction and Filtration

These areas are discussed in chapters 11 and 12. Their effect on density, however, can be stated relatively simply. Primary beam restriction is achieved

TABLE 8–6	BASIC GRID CONVERSION RATIOS FOR CHANGING FROM NON-GRID TO GRID TECHNIQUE		
NON-GRID TO GRID*	**WHEN mAs USE IS INCREASED**	**WHEN kVp USE IS INCREASED**	**MAXIMUM kVp FOR GRID RATIO**
5:1	2 × original mAs	+ 8 kVp	80
8:1	4 × original mAs	+ 20 kVp	90–100
12:1	5 × original mAs	+ 25 kVp	110–120
16:1	6 × original mAs	+ 30 kVp	150

*Note that kVp increases may be preferable to mAs increases when technique is changed from non-grid exposure to grid exposure. An increase in mAs reduces contrast as well as increases exposure time, whereas an increase in kVp does not increase radiation dosage. Also, unless the kVp is excessive, decreasing mAs permits the penetration value of the total exposure to be retained.

by the use of collimators, diaphragms, and occasionally cones, Figure 8-16. The purpose of these devices is to minimize the amount of scattered radiation that reaches the film. An increase in scattered radiation reaching the film results in fog, which causes an increase in density and a resultant decrease in contrast. The primary beam should be limited or confined to the area of the structure being radiographed, leaving only a narrow border within the edges of the film. The beam must at least be confined to the size of the film itself. Unnecessarily exposing large areas beyond the film edges results in added density in the radiographic image and increased dosage to the patient.

Filtration

Filtration is the process of filtering the beam of radiation through some type of material that will remove lower-energy radiation from the beam and prevent them from reaching the patient. The filter should be a type of material that will allow the more useful higher-energy radiation to pass through unchanged, but will absorb nonuseful lower-energy radiation. Aluminum is a material of choice for filters because it is less expensive than other mate-

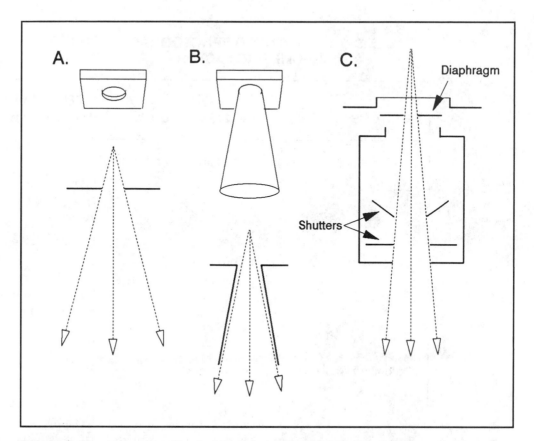

Figure 8-16. A) A sheet of lead with a hole in the center (aperture diaphragm). B) A sheet of metal or lead (diaphragm) with a cylinder cone attached. The lead is placed close to the radiation source with the cone extending down. The length and diameter of the cone determine the size of the field exposed. C) A collimator with multiple shutters. The shutters are variable by external controls, but generally are set on automatic field size. Near the tube window is a diaphragm designed to minimize off-focus radiation. The collimator is used for positive beam limitation (PBL) as required by law.

rials and as it absorbs lower-energy radiation well while allowing passage of higher-energy radiation. The aluminum is placed within the beam, either at the tube-window aperture or at the collimator opening. This is called added filtration and may measure 2.0 mm of aluminum or its equivalent. There is usually 0.5 mm of filtration within the tube itself, made up by the glass tube and its surrounding insulating oil. This is called inherent (built-in) filtration. The total minimal amount of beam filtration should be about 2.5 mm (inherent and added) of aluminum equivalent. If there were no

TABLE 8–7 SUMMARY OF PHOTOGRAPHIC AND GEOMETRIC FACTORS

FACTORS	CONTROLLED BY	INFLUENCED/ AFFECTED BY
Photographic Factors		
Density	mAs	SID Heel effect kVp Fog processing
Contrast	Kilovoltage	Filters Fog (all forms) Film processing Subject contrast Type of film Pathology
Secondary Radiation Fog		Size of area exposed Compression Cones Diaphragms Grids kVp
Geometric Factors		
Recorded Detail		Focal-spot size Object-film distance Motion Screen-crystal size Film-screen contact
Image Size (Magnification)		Focus-film distance Object-film distance
Image Size (Distortion)		Alignment of tube to film Alignment of part to film Object-film distance

added filtration to the radiation beam and lower-energy radiation were permitted to reach the film, the radiographic image density and patient dosage would increase. For medical radiography, patient dosage is therefore most effectively reduced with 2.5 mm of total filtration.

Processing

Three processing related elements can adversely affect film density if they are not appropriately managed. These are *safelights*, *film age*, and *chemicals*. Although these are discussed in detail in chapter 9, a brief review is needed here. The following three requirements may be properly set by following the recommendations of the film manufacturer: 1) the safelight must have the correct color of filter for the type(s) of film used; 2) it must have the correct size (wattage) bulb; and 3) it must be placed at the correct distance from the film-loading area and processor.

Age of film is important. Film comes from the manufacturer with an expiration date. Film boxes should be stored so that the oldest film is always used prior to that more recently dated.

Processor chemicals are precisely controlled by a time-temperature processing method. Any increase in the temperature is likely to add density to the film. Also, if the chemicals are not properly replenished and become exhausted or contaminated for any reason, added chemical density will occur on the film. All of the above, if not controlled, will create fog on the film that will result in increased density.

SUMMARY

A summary of photographic factors and geometric factors appears in Table 8-7.

REVIEW QUESTIONS

1. Radiographic density is best defined as the
   a) sharpness of the radiographic image
   b) distortion of the image shape and size
   c) degree of blackness in the radiograph
   d) degree of difference between the light and dark areas
2. Radiographic contrast is best defined as the
   a) sharpness of the radiographic image
   b) distortion of the image shape and size
   c) degree of blackness in the radiograph
   d) degree of difference between the light and dark areas

3. Select the exposure setting that will result in the greatest density:

	mA	TIME	SID
a)	100	1/2 second	36"
b)	200	1/4 second	30"
c)	300	1/6 second	40"
d)	400	1/8 second	46"

4. To apply heel effect when radiographing a femur, position the thicker anatomic part beneath the
   a) cathode
   b) anode
   c) cathode or anode
   d) there is little difference

5. A sharp difference between the light and dark areas of a radiographic image is termed
   a) subject contrast
   b) long-scale contrast
   c) short-scale contrast
   d) inherent contrast

6. To change from a short-scale contrast to a long-scale contrast
   a) decrease mAs and increase kVp
   b) decrease mAs and decrease kVp
   c) increase mAs and decrease kVp
   d) increase mAs and increase kVp

7. A grid should be used when the body part being radiographed is
   a) likely to produce motion
   b) thicker than twelve centimeters
   c) subject to variations in size
   d) radiolucent

8. Which of the following technical factor sets is likely to result in the greatest amount of magnification?

	mAs	OFD	SID
a)	30	6"	36"
b)	50	5"	50"
c)	75	4"	60"
d)	100	3"	72"

9. The photographic properties of a radiograph consist of the following elements:
   a) recorded detail
   b) density and contrast
   c) magnification and distortion
   d) a and b
   e) a and c

10. The primary purpose of a grid is to reduce the effects of _____ on the image.
    a) density
    b) contrast
    c) scattered radiation
    d) all of the above

11. When any of several combinations of mA and T will produce an equivalent amount of mAs, the result is called
    a) Ohm's Law
    b) reciprocity law
    c) inverse square law
    d) none of the above

12. Heat unit (HU) capacity is determined by the following formula:
    a) mA × T
    b) mA × kVp
    c) mA × T × kVp
    d) mA × T × kVp²

13. *The intensity of radiation is inversely proportional to the square of the distance* expresses the relationship between:
    a) distance and density
    b) distance and contrast
    c) distance and focal-spot size
    d) distance and radiation intensity

14. A change in SID from an original position of 40″ to an increased position of 60″ will change the following effect of _____ .
    a) density (mA)
    b) intensity (SID)
    c) penetration (kVp)
    d) all of the above

15. The term "geometric blur" or penumbra is associated with the effects of the following factor(s):
    a) FSS
    b) SID
    c) OFD
    d) a and c
    e) a, b, c

Radiographic Film Processing

CHAPTER OUTLINE

OBJECTIVES

Upon completion of the chapter, the student will meet the following objectives by verifying knowledge, facts, and principles presented through oral and written communication at a level deemed competent and will meet the task objectives by demonstrating the specific behavior as identified in the terminal performance objectives of the procedures.

1. Identify appropriate responses related to processing area location, construction, and function.
2. Describe the composition of screen film and explain the function of each part.
3. Recall three characteristics of screen film.
4. Identify proper procedures for handling and storing radiographic film.
5. Outline the procedure for checking safelight illumination.
6. Explain the purpose of intensifying screens.
7. Identify the difference between calcium-tungstate and rare-earth screens.
8. Outline the procedure for proper care and cleaning of intensifying screens.
9. Discuss the basic difference between manual and automatic processing.
10. Describe the steps in film processing.
11. Explain the purpose of replenishment of processing chemicals.
12. Recognize common film artifacts and identify causative factors.
13. Demonstrate competence in each task listed. Refer to the appendix for the individual procedure/performance guides.

TASKS:

9-1 Testing safelight performance
9-2 Maintaining master card file or computer system
9-3 Indexing and filing radiographs
9-4 Processing loans of radiographs
9-5 Loading and unloading a cassette
9-6 Cleaning intensifying screens
9-7 Testing cassette for screen-film contact
9-8 Processing film by manual method
9-9 Processing film by automatic method

INTRODUCTION

"Film processing can make or break an otherwise perfect radiograph." This statement, common among radiographers, refers to the importance of film processing in the production of diagnostic radiographs. For proper film processing to occur, many tasks must be completed. This starts with a well-maintained darkroom environment, equipment, and supplies and ends with a fully processed diagnostic radiograph.

This chapter introduces theory about maintaining the darkroom environment, film and screen construction and proper care, film processing, and the interrelated factors involved in producing diagnostic-quality radiographs.

PROCESSING AREA CONSIDERATIONS

A processing area should offer an environment in which the necessary functions can be carried out safely and efficiently, without providing hazards that would compromise the diagnostic quality of finished radiographs. The processing area actually requires "safe" artificial light rather than total blackness. However, the processing area is still commonly called "the darkroom," and this term will be used throughout the chapter.

Location of the Darkroom

Whether they are located in an office or in a hospital, most processing areas today are automated. To save time, darkrooms are generally located near the radiographic rooms. The distance of the darkroom from the radiography rooms is more important in a multi-doctor clinic or large hospital, where the patient volume may require a full-time person to perform film processing and equipment maintenance.

Darkroom ventilation should provide a constant flow of fresh air with a temperature between 70° F and 80° F. The relative humidity level should be maintained at between 50 percent and 60 percent. This prevents a buildup of chemical odors, yet allows enough air moisture to prevent static electricity that can discharge to the film and cause artifacts. A well-ventilated darkroom is also important for a healthy work environment. A film-viewing area may be adjacent to the darkroom where radiographs can be viewed, Figure 9-1. The darkroom should be large enough to provide space for loading and unloading cassettes, film storage bin, processing equipment, and related accessories.

Walls adjacent to the radiographic rooms should be shielded with 1.6 mm (1/16 in) lead all the way to the ceiling to protect unexposed film from radiation exposure. Passboxes may be built into the walls to allow passage of cassettes between the darkroom and radiographic room. A typical passbox has two sets of doors to allow such passage between rooms and an interlock

Figure 9-1. Sketch of typical darkroom arrangement with essential areas identified

Figure 9-2. Passbox located between darkroom and radiographic room. Note double-lock doors and easy accessibility to film-loading bench. *(Reprinted courtesy of Eastman Kodak Company)*

system on each set of doors to prevent accidental light exposure should both be opened at the same time, Figure 9-2. Each set of doors will have two compartments, one for exposed and one for unexposed cassettes. The ideal location for a passbox is near the film-loading bench in the darkroom.

Darkroom walls and floor should be covered with a non-porous, chemical- and stain-resistant surface (e.g., Formica®). A radiographic processing area should have a single entrance door that allows for absolute lighttight fittings. Variations on the single entrance are: 1) a maze-type entry, Figure 9-3; 2) a revolving door, Figure 9-4; and 3) an electric interlocking door system. Whatever the entrance design, the purpose is to protect radiographic film from being struck by light and/or radiation and being fogged. Processing-area lighting consists of safelight, radiographic illumination, and regular lighting.

RADIOGRAPHIC FILM

A radiograph is a permanent image created when ionizing radiation passes through matter and onto photographic film. The image is latent, or invisible,

Figure 9-3. Darkroom with maze entrance

Figure 9-4. Revolving darkroom door. The outer rim is built into the wall and has two openings: one into the darkroom and one to the outside. The door's inner rim is suspended, which allows it to rotate on a central bearing. The inner rim's opening can be turned to coincide with the outer rim's openings.

and will become manifest, or visible, after the film is processed. The recording medium, or radiographic film, plays a very critical role in the production of diagnostic radiographs. If the film is defective, or has been improperly stored or handled, the final diagnostic image may be less than perfect. Also, many things can happen during the film-processing stage that may detract from the diagnostic value of the radiograph. To avoid these problems, it is helpful to learn about radiographic film construction, latent image formation, types of film, and proper film handling and storage.

Radiographic film consists of two parts, the base and the emulsion, surrounded by a protective covering of gelatin called the supercoating. The base is constructed of a polyester that provides a rigid yet flexible support for the emulsion. A subcoating of adhesive covers the base and serves to bind the emulsion to the base polyester. The emulsion consists of a mixture of gelatin and silver halide crystals. Usually, 95 percent of the silver halide consists of silver bromide with the remainder being silver iodide.

Most radiographic film is coated on both sides and thus is called double emulsion film. The emulsion is the most important layer of the film because it contains the crystals that will hold the latent image formation. The gelatin in the emulsion allows for an even distribution of the silver halide crystals.

Its properties allow for rapid softening in the developer solution and quick hardening in the fixer solution. Refer to Figure 9-5, a cross section of radiographic film. The emulsion reaction to ionizing radiation can be altered by the way the crystals are manufactured and their mixture. Each manufacturer of film closely guards the unique formulas that are responsible for its film characteristics. Film characteristics include speed, contrast, and resolution. Each of these areas will be included in the discussion on film types.

Latent Image Formation

As ionizing radiation exits from matter and strikes radiographic film, energy is deposited in the emulsion. The transfer of information between the radiation and film emulsion is by photoelectric interaction. Each silver halide crystal has on its surface sensitive specks of tiny particles of atomic silver and silver sulfide. When these specks are struck by ionizing radiation, ionization of the silver halide crystals results in charged silver ions and negatively charged bromine ions, expressed as:

$$AgBr + X\text{-rays} \rightarrow Ag^+ + Br^-$$

These sensitized specks will react to the developer chemicals during film processing. Silver halide crystals that have been ionized (irradiated) will be changed into black grains through the development process. Silver halide

Figure 9-5. Cross section of radiographic film

crystals that have not been ionized will remain in crystal form and will not be changed during the development stage of film processing. These unexposed, undeveloped silver halide crystals will react to the fixer chemicals and will be released from the emulsion in the fixation step of processing and recovered through a silver-recovery chamber.

Types of X-ray Film

Many different types of film are manufactured for medical radiography. This variety reflects the diversity of radiographic procedures requiring special application film, such as those used in mammography, cardiography, dental radiography, and so forth. Limited radiographers will generally use only the two common types of X-ray films, screen-type film and direct exposure film (often called nonscreen film). The major differences between the two types of film are the thickness of the film emulsion and whether it responds to both X ray and light emitted from the intensifying screen.

Direct exposure film responds best to X-ray. Direct exposure film is rarely used today because (1) its increased emulsion silver content makes it more costly and (2) it requires a much higher X-ray exposure. *Because direct exposure film requires an increase in X-ray exposure, its use does not justify the increase in radiation exposure to the patient*. By using screen-type film, the radiation exposure to the patient can be reduced. This is possible because screen film (sensitive to light) is used with intensifying screens that emit light during the X-ray exposure, thereby allowing a reduction in the X-ray exposure.

Screen film has three characteristics that are routinely considered: contrast (high or low), speed (sensitivity), and light absorption. Each film manufacturer produces screen film with a certain level of contrast. This level may be high-contrast, which produces a very black-and-white shaded image, or low-contrast, which produces a gray shaded image. The film contrast of a particular brand of film is directly related to the latitude or range of exposure factors (mA, time, kVp) that will produce an acceptable image. Usually film manufacturers provide two or more latitudes, referred to as medium- or high-contrast film. The physician who is responsible for interpreting the radiographic image may wish to select the level of film contrast to be used for most radiographic procedures.

Screen film is also available in different speeds or sensitivity. The speed of a screen film refers to how fast the silver halide crystals in the emulsion respond to the light emitted from the intensifying screens. High-speed (fast) screen film contains a thick emulsion, large crystals, or a higher concentration of crystals in the emulsion. Visibility of anatomic detail on the finished radiograph may be decreased with the use of high-speed (fast) screen film. An advantage, however, of this type of film is the faster exposure times can be used. Film-speed and contrast-level selection should be a collective effort of the radiographer and physician.

Spectral absorption, commonly called spectral matching, refers to the use of film whose sensitivity is correctly matched to the light spectrum emitted from the intensifying screen. Calcium-tungstate intensifying screens emit blue and blue violet light and should be matched to silver halide emulsion film or blue-sensitive film. Rare-earth intensifying screens should be matched to screen film that is sensitive to green light. However, they may also be compatible with blue-sensitive film. Correct spectral matching is also referred to as film-screen combination or spectral system. Selecting the correct combination is very important because if the match is incorrect, the film will not respond properly and the patient may receive more radiation than necessary because of incorrect exposure that may result in a repeat radiograph.

Because X-ray film is sensitive to light, the lamps or safelights used in the darkroom must meet certain requirements. Darkroom lamps are used to provide a minimum of light to allow the operator some illumination. Because exposed screen film is approximately eight times more sensitive to light than unexposed film, safelights must have their light filtered. For blue-sensitive film, an amber (Wratten 6-B) light generally is used. An amber filter will only allow light having wavelengths longer than 550 mm or beyond the spectral response of blue-sensitive film to be emitted. A reddish brown filter is used with green-sensitive film and can also be used with blue-sensitive film. Safelights should be installed at least three feet from the area where the film will be handled and processed. Light bulb wattage in the safelight should not exceed the manufacturer's recommendations for the specific type filter.

Safelights are designed for either indirect ceiling illumination or direct illumination. One way to determine whether a safelight is actually safe is to check the safelight illumination, evaluate the results, and take necessary action if an unsafe condition exists. Remember that safelight illumination as well as light leaks into the darkroom area and can cause fog or an undesirable film darkening that decreases the diagnostic value of the radiograph. It is important to periodically check the safelight filter for cracks and light leaks in the lamp (filter) housing. Exercise 9-1 in the appendix will help you practice how to test safelight performance.

Film Identification

Patient identification, date, right or left marker, and other data can be permanently marked on a radiograph. Two common methods of identification are: (1) attaching lead markers to the cassette before the exposure is made, Figure 9-6A and (2) a photographic transfer of data, Figure 9-6B. Generally,

Figure 9-6A. Film identification markers

Figure 9-6B. Photographic transferring of patient information to the radiograph *(Reprinted courtesy of Eastman Kodak Company)*

both methods are used. The lead marker contains the patient's identification number, date, a right or left letter, and the doctor or facility name. The photographic marker usually contains more detailed data such as the patient's address, sex, age, religion, insurance identification, etc., Figure 9-7.

In the photographic method of identification, a card containing the patient data is inserted into a camera device. With the white lights off, the exposed radiograph is placed in the camera window, and a very quick light exposure is made, thereby transferring the patient data to the film, Figure 9-8. Cassettes

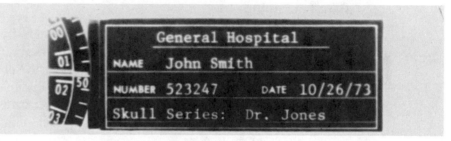

Figure 9-7. Identification information as it appears on radiograph *(Reprinted courtesy of Eastman Kodak Company)*

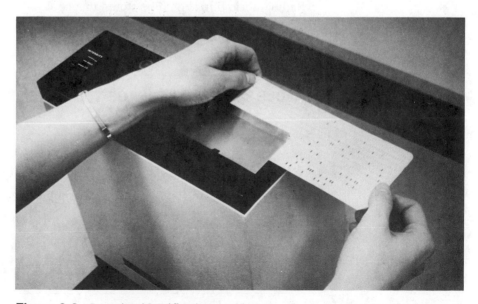

Figure 9-8. Inserting identification card into top of camera *(Reprinted courtesy of Eastman Kodak Company)*

used with this method of identification must have a lead blocker that protects the area of the film that will later be imprinted with patient data.

RADIOGRAPHIC-FILM STORAGE AND HANDLING

Radiographic film is sensitive to X rays, heat, light, chemical fumes, moisture, pressure, and any kind of rough handling, i.e., bending, scratching, crimping, etc. Radiographic film must be properly stored and carefully handled to ensure that damage does not occur.

Film Packaging

Radiographic film is packaged in a moisture-free, sealed bag with cardboard supports. The bag is packaged in a heavy duty plastic bag within a sealed cardboard shipping carton. The outside of the carton indicates the type of film, quantity, and expiration date. Film is available in quantities of twenty-five, fifty, and one hundred sheets per carton. Individually wrapped sheets of film can also be purchased; such film is called interleaved or prewrapped film.

Film Storage

Radiographic film should be stored in a cool, dry place. The temperature

TABLE 9–1	FILM STORAGE TEMPERATURE/TIME LENGTH USABLE RELATIONSHIPS
MAINTAINED STORAGE TEMPERATURE	**APPROXIMATE LENGTH OF TIME FILM USABLE**
90–100°F	2–3 days
70°F	2 months
60°F	6 months
50°F	1 year

of the storage area has a direct influence on the length of time unexposed film can be maintained and used (refer to Table 9-1). The best temperature for film storage is between 60° F and 70° F and 40 percent and 50 percent relative humidity. Stored film should also be protected from x-radiation, fumes, chemicals, and any gas-producing substance. Film boxes should never be subjected to excessive pressure. To avoid pressure marks, warping, and bending, boxes of unexposed film should always be stored upright.

Stored film should be used prior to the expiration date. Stored film boxes should be rotated as new shipments arrive. Rotate the stock so that film with a close expiration date is always used first. This avoids having to discard expired film and saves money in film expense.

Once a film box is opened, a film bin, Figure 9-9, provides ideal storage. A film bin has separate compartments to hold different film sizes and is usually installed beneath the film loading area. Film bins may be electrically connected to the overhead lights. In this case, the lights will not turn on if the film bin drawer is open. Also, the darkroom entrance door may be electrically connected to the film bin to prevent accidental light exposure to the film should the door be opened while the bin is open.

Film fog is defined as an undesirable increase in the density of the emulsion, either before or after radiation exposure. The additional film density or fog decreases the quality of the radiographic image by reducing the visibility of the diagnostic information. Light is only one of several causes of fog. Refer to Table 9-2 for a brief listing of the causes of fog.

Figure 9-9. Film bin. A film bin is generally installed in existing counter space.

TABLE 9–2   CAUSES OF FILM FOG

SOURCE	PRECAUTION TO AVOID
Chemical Fumes	Certain chemical fumes will cause the emulsion to become fogged. Do not store films in an area that contains chemical fumes and is poorly ventilated.
Temperature and Humidity	Store films in an area with 40–50 percent relative humidity and constant temperature range between 60–70° F.
Radiation	Film must be stored in an area where it is protected from radiation. Stored film must be protected from primary and secondary scatter radiation.
Pressure	Store film boxes on edge, never stack them. Avoid dropping film boxes.
Age	Use film before the expiration date indicated on the film box. Rotate stock.

Film Handling

X-ray film must be handled carefully to avoid extraneous marks and images on the radiograph; such marks or images are called artifacts. An artifact can also be defined as an area of increased or decreased film darkening or density. Handle film carefully avoiding creasing or bending and rapid movement of the film, which can cause static electric discharges to be conveyed to the film, Figure 9-10. Proper loading and unloading of cassettes and direct exposure film envelopes are essential.

When films are carelessly handled by an individual loading and unloading cassettes, the films may be bent. This damages the emulsion and results in artifacts called crescent or crinkle marks, semicircular in shape. A white crescent-shaped mark results from bending the film before exposure. A black crescent-shaped mark is caused from bending the film after it has been exposed.

Figure 9-10. Artifacts resulting from static electric discharges to the film

Film should also always be handled with clean, oil-free, and dry hands. Film-handling errors are one cause of film artifacts. For further information on film artifacts, refer to the "film processing" section of this chapter.

Maintaining Radiographic Film

Processed radiographs are a permanent, legal patient record and should be stored at 60° to 70° F temperature and 40–50 percent relative humidity. The storage area should be free of chemical fumes, moisture, and excessive changes in temperature or humidity.

Each facility establishes a particular protocol for film filing and retrieval. It is important that the system provide quick access to the records as needed.

Film filing folders should be made of materials that do not contain chemicals that can react with the stored radiographs. There are many ways to file and maintain radiographs. Exercises 9-2 and 9-3 in the appendix illustrate procedures that are only two of many possible methods in current use today.

Each facility will also determine how to handle requests for loans of radiographs. One example would include information on who may request films, whether a written request is required, and if all or only the most recent radiographs are provided. Rather than loan original radiographs, a facility may provide duplicates at a nominal charge. Duplication of radiographs allows the facility to maintain a complete record, yet share the information with others providing medical care to the same patient. Exercise 9-4 in the appendix outlines a suggested protocol for loaning radiographs.

INTENSIFYING SCREENS

In 1895, German physicist Wilhelm Conrad Roentgen was operating a vacuum tube when he noticed a glow coming from a cardboard coated with a chemical, barium platinocyanide. The vacuum tube was covered so that no light escaped, yet the glow or fluorescence from the cardboard seemed to intensify when it was moved closer to the tube. Roentgen called his discovery "x-radiation" and began to investigate its properties further. In 1901, Roentgen won the first Nobel prize in physics for his discovery. His investigation led not only to the discovery and application of x-radiation but also to the use of chemically coated fluorescent screens in radiography.

The very thing that makes x-rays useful—their penetrating power—also makes them difficult to record. For example, of the x-ray intensity in the primary beam emerging from the patient, only about 1 or 2 percent is absorbed by a sheet of x-ray film and 98 percent or more is wasted. Early in the history of x-rays, the need to use more of this wasted x-ray energy was recognized. This led to the coating of photosensitive emulsion on both sides of the x-ray plate, doubling the absorption of the single-coated material. It also led to the introduction of fluorescent intensifying screens.[1]

Since less than 2 percent of the X rays produced are absorbed by the film emulsion, the light emitted by the intensifying screens increase the effect on the emulsion, thereby allowing a decrease in X-ray exposure to the patient. In the last decade, the most dramatic reductions in radiation exposure to patients have resulted from the introduction of intensifying screens that have rare-earth phosphors capable of emitting even greater amounts of light.

Intensifying screens look like thin sheets of plastic. They are available in sizes corresponding to film sizes. Screens are mounted inside cassettes. Screens, like radiographic film, consist of layers, each having a specific purpose. Most intensifying screens have four layers: protective coating, phosphor, reflective layer, and base, Figure 9-11.

The protective coating is the outermost layer of the screen and is closest to the film. This coating is transparent and serves to reduce abrasion that would damage the screen surface. It also reduces the accumulation of static electricity. This protective surface may be cleaned without causing damage to the active fluorescent phosphor.

The phosphor, or active layer, is responsible for emitting light when struck by X rays. Another way of expressing this phenomenon is to say that the phosphor is responsible for converting the energy of the X-ray beam into visible light. Phosphors used in screens may be crystalline calcium tungstate, zinc sulfide, barium lead sulfate, or the rare earths gadolinium, lanthanum, and yttrium. Today, however, calcium tungstate or the rare earths are most

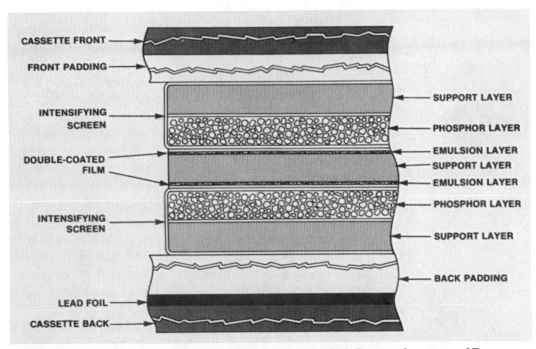

Figure 9-11. Loaded cassette with the four layers identified *(Reprinted courtesy of Eastman Kodak Company)*

commonly in use. Although rare-earth phosphor screens are more costly, they are the phosphor most often used. The major advantage of rare-earth screens over conventional calcium-tungstate screens is speed. Since rare-earth screens are faster, they require less X-ray exposure to the patient. Differences in intensifying screens result from the differences in the phosphor composition, concentration, and crystal size.

For a phosphor to be used in an intensifying screen, it must have the following properties:

1. A high atomic number allowing for greater X-ray interaction with the phosphor
2. A high *conversion efficiency*, or the ability to emit a great amount of light
3. *Spectral matching*, meaning that the light emitted is of a wavelength (color) to match the sensitivity of the X-ray film
4. Should not continue to flow or emit light after the X-ray interaction stops. *Phosphorescence* is the continued emission of light by the phosphor after the exposure has ended. This is often referred to as screen afterglow or screen lag.

The reflective layer of the screen is between the phosphor and the base. The reflective layer keeps the light emitted by the phosphors directed toward the film.

The purpose of the base layer of the screen is to provide support for the phosphor layer. It consists of a tough polyester that is chemically inert, flexible, and resists damage from the radiation.

Intensifying screens have characteristics that are important to the limited radiographer. These characteristics include intensification factor (screen speed) and resolution. The intensification factor measures the speed of the screen. Screen speed is defined simply as the screen's ability to produce density with a given exposure to X rays. There are three major speed categories of calcium-tungstate screens: medium speed, high speed, and fine detail (slow) speed. Rare-earth screens can be up to twelve hundred times faster than the categories listed for calcium-tungstate screens. Generally, these categories are described by comparing one against the others. Screen speed cannot be accurately measured, so in most discussions, the speeds will be compared in relation to their use and results.

The higher the speed of the screen, the more density will be produced at a given exposure. Use of high-speed screens reduces radiation exposure to the patient. This is possible because a greater intensification (more light) is produced by the high-speed screen, therefore, less exposure is needed to produce an image.

Although medium- and fine-detail-speed screens are available, most limited radiographers will use high-speed screens or rare-earth screens. Medium- and fine-detail-speed screens are used for specialty radiography when increased visibility of anatomic detail is desired. However, the patient may receive more radiation exposure with medium- and fine-detail-speed screens than with fast-speed screens or rare-earth screens.

Resolution is another important characteristic of intensifying screens. It is defined as the ability of a system to consistently produce an image of an object. To demonstrate resolution, one might look through a camera lens. If the object being viewed is out of focus, it has poor resolution. A rule of thumb to remember about screen resolution is that those conditions that increase the intensification factor reduce resolution. This means that high-speed screens with their large-size phosphor crystals will have a lower resolution than fine detail screens. Resolution increases as the phosphor crystals become smaller and the phosphor layer thinner. As previously mentioned, one can increase resolution with fine detail screens; however, the patient radiation exposure increases because these screens require more exposure than do fast-speed or rare-earth screens.

The choice of a film-screen combination, or film-imaging system, can significantly affect the patient's radiation exposure and the diagnostic quality of the radiation. A rule to follow regarding the selection of film and screens is to use the type and speed of film for the particular screen (e.g., high-speed film with a high-speed intensifying screen).

Direct Exposure or Cassette

Two types of film holders are used for radiography examinations: a direct exposure holder or a cassette that contains intensifying screens. Both film-holding devices will be discussed; however, direct exposure film holders are rarely used because of the increase in exposure required. Because cassettes contain a pair of intensifying screens that light up when struck by radiation, the patient's exposure dose is less than is required by a direct exposure holder containing no intensifying screens.

A direct exposure film holder, commonly called a "cardboard," is a light-proof envelope. Direct exposure (nonscreen) film is used with this type of film holder. These holders have a radiographic tube side that must face the tube during the exposure and a back side lined with lead foil to prevent scatter radiation from striking the film. Direct film holders are used for radiography of thin body parts measuring less than twelve centimeters. The advantage of direct exposure is that it provides good resolution or detail of the image. This results from the direct information transfer to the film as compared to the intensification factor of intensifying screens where some detail is lost as a result of the delay in light emitted by the crystal phosphors. *Today, however, the potential benefit of direct exposure cannot be justified because of the increase in radiation exposure required as compared to using a cassette.*

A cassette is a rigid holder containing intensifying screens. The front surface, or tube side, is made of thin, yet sturdy, plastic. The back of the cassette provides some type of spring closure device to maintain an even pressure on the film when the holder is closed. Attached to the inside are the front and back intensifying screens. A compression material such as felt is installed between each screen and the cassette cover. This material serves to further provide a good film-screen contact when the cassette is closed. Proper film loading and unloading is important in maintaining the surface of the screen as well as the condition of the film. Exercise 9-5 in the appendix will help you learn how to properly load and unload film from a cassette.

The outside of a cassette may be cleaned with a disinfectant as frequently as necessary. The intensifying screens, however, require regular inspection and cleaning. Care must be taken to keep the screens dry and to avoid stains and scratches that may cause permanent damage. Common types of soiling are from blood, lipstick, hair dressing, and processing solutions. Foreign objects, such as small pieces of paper, hair, etc., can also find their way into a cassette. Static electricity can cause dust particles to be attracted to the screen. Many commercial screen-cleaning solutions include an antistatic compound to reduce static electricity.

Always remember the important contribution of light energy that intensifying screens make to the formation of the latent image. With this in mind, it is easy to understand that any stain, soil, or matter on the screen surface can interfere with the amount of light reaching the film. An object or stain on a screen surface will appear as an unwanted shadow or artifact on the finished radiograph.

Keeping cassettes closed and properly stored away from moisture will help to avoid damage to the intensifying screens. This also protects the screen's phosphors from light, which can weaken the chemical fluorescence of the phosphor.

A cassette that is closed and latched is assumed to be loaded with unexposed film. If, at any time, a cassette must be closed and latched without film, identify it with a note stating that it is unloaded. This precaution will help to avoid a repeat examination and unnecessary radiation exposure to a patient.

Good darkroom housekeeping to keep the darkroom and film-loading areas clean is essential. Screens should be cleaned according to the manufacturer's instructions, which often recommend a specific commercial cleaning solution. Also, cleaning solutions for calcium-tungstate screens may not be suitable for rare-earth screens because of optical residue that can interfere with the light emission. The frequency at which intensifying screens are cleaned depends upon a number of factors: manufacturer's suggested cleaning schedule, amount of use the screens receive, and overall cleanliness of the darkroom environment and operator. Exercise 9-6 in the appendix is a sample procedure for cleaning intensifying screens.

Screen-Film Contact

Intensifying screens must be in direct contact with the film across its entire surface. Poor screen-film contact results in a severe loss of recorded detail and a slight decrease in density on the finished radiograph. The compression material (such as felt) and metal backings on the cassette are responsible for proper screen-film contact, Figure 9-12. As a result of constant use or abuse, the compression material, spring latches, or backing may become warped. When this happens, even pressure is not exerted on the screens, which causes poor screen-film contact. Other factors that can contribute to poor screen-film contact are: (1) air trapped between screen and film, (2) foreign matter on the screen surface, and (3) improperly mounted screens. The loss of screen-film contact may be gradual, and for this reason, the contact should be checked on a regular basis. Exercise 9-7 in the appendix provides practice in checking for poor screen-film contact.

FILM PROCESSING

Chemical processing changes the latent image held in the film emulsion into a manifest image. In the early days of radiography, film processing was done manually, by moving the film from the developer to the fixer tank by hand. Drying of the radiograph was accomplished by the clothesline method of air drying. Needless to say, manual processing was not always a precise procedure and often did not allow for consistent processing results. Today, most medical facilities have automatic film processors; however, a brief section will be included on manual processing because many small medical

A

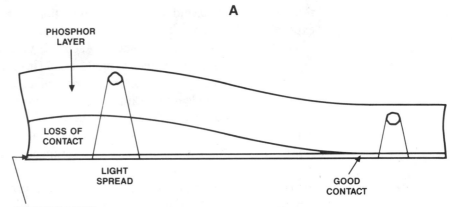

PHOSPHOR
LAYER

LOSS OF
CONTACT

LIGHT
SPREAD

GOOD
CONTACT

EMULSION LAYER

B

Figure 9-12. Test for screen-film contact. A) Diagram showing loss of screen-film contact; B) Radiograph showing effect of poor screen-film contact. *(Reprinted courtesy of Eastman Kodak Company)*

clinics may still use this method. The basic steps of film processing are similar for automatic and manual processing: development, fixation, wash, and drying processes. The chemicals used in each method are similar, except that the strength concentration is higher for automatic processor chemistry.

Also, of course, automatic processing involves higher solution temperatures and shorter processing times.

Overview of Film-Processing Steps

Each step will be discussed in greater detail, but it helps to form a mental image of the steps required to process a radiograph. After the cassette is unloaded in the darkroom, the exposed film is ready to be developed. The developer is responsible for converting the exposed silver halide crystals into metallic silver. The fixer actually performs two important functions: it removes the unexposed and undeveloped silver halide crystals from the emulsion and hardens the soft gelatin. The washing process removes fixer solution from the film emulsion. Drying the radiograph prepares it for viewing and later storage.

Processing Solutions

Tables 9-3 and 9-4 list the chemical ingredients of the developer and fixer.

Preparation of Solutions

Preparation of solutions is a very important step in processing. Chemical solutions should be prepared according to the manufacturer's directions and safety specifications. The following general precautions are reprinted from the *Fundamentals of Radiography*, 12th edition.[2]

General Precautions. It is extremely important to avoid chemical contamination of processing solutions because minute quantities of impurities can produce undesirable effects. Therefore:

1. Clean tanks and covers thoroughly before starting to mix fresh solutions.
2. Be careful not to splash ingredients of one solution into another. For example, small amounts of fixer can significantly change developer behavior. Be sure to use splash guards and drip trays when removing or installing processor racks because solutions can drip and contaminate other chemical tanks.
3. Use mixing and storage containers made of corrosion-resistant materials (enamel, hard-glazed earthenware, polyethylene, polypropylene, glass, hard rubber, ANSI Type 316 stainless steel with 2 to 3 percent molybdenum). Never use containers made of reactive materials such as tin, copper, zinc, aluminum, or galvanized iron.

TABLE 9–3 DEVELOPER CHEMISTRY

SOLVENT	Water	Dissolves the developer chemicals and causes gelatin in film emulsion to swell
DEVELOPING AGENTS	Phenidone (automatic processing) Elon and hydroquinone (manual processing)	Converts exposed silver halide crystals into metallic silver
ACCELERATORS	Sodium or potassium hydroxide	An alkali added to the developer to increase the chemical activity
PRESERVATIVES	Sodium sulfite	Prevents oxidation
RESTRAINERS	Potassium bromide Potassium iodide	Controls activity of reducing agents and prevents chemical fog
HARDENER	Glutaraldehyde	**ONLY** used for automatic processing; controls swelling of the emulsion

TABLE 9–4 FIXER CHEMISTRY

SOLVENT	Water	Dissolves the fixer chemicals
CLEARING AND FIXING AGENTS	Ammonium thiosulfate (Hypo)	Dissolves and removes undeveloped silver halide crystals and changes the unexposed areas of the film from milky to clear and translucent
PRESERVATIVES	Sodium sulfite	Prevents decomposition of the clearing agents
HARDENER	Aluminum chloride or Potassium alum	Shrinks and hardens the emulsion
ACIDIFIER	Acetic acid	Provides an acid pH and neutralizes the alkaline developer
BUFFER		Chemicals added to fixing solution to stabilize and balance the acid-alkaline pH of the solutions

4. Do not use tanks or other containers that have been soldered because the reaction of the solution with the solder metals causes chemical fog on film.
5. Cover solution tanks when not in use to keep out dirt and reduce the rate of oxidation and evaporation. The tank cover can either fit over the top or float on the solution.
6. Use two stirring paddles or plungers—one for the developer and one for the fixer. Identify and keep them separate for each solution. After use, wash them in warm water and hang them up to dry.
7. Be very careful if mercury thermometers are used for measuring solution temperatures. If such a thermometer is broken, the mercury is hazardous because of its toxicity. Also, mercury can produce a high fog level on film.
8. Finally, adjust the temperature of the water in which the chemicals are to be dissolved as recommended on package labels.[3]

Processing chemicals are available in dry and liquid form. It is important to follow the manufacturer's directions for mixing chemicals. Some general precautions include:

1. Dry chemicals should be mixed away from stored film.
2. Liquid chemicals should be mixed with water of the same temperature.
3. All chemicals should be thoroughly stirred while mixing.
4. Follow recommended safety precautions regarding inhaling chemical vapors or dry particles and eye and skin contact when using processing chemicals.

As in any chemical reaction, optimum conditions of time, temperature, and strength of solutions are critical to the process. It is best to purchase processing chemicals that are compatible to the film because the manufacturer's recommendations regarding ideal conditions can be followed to the letter. Like film-screen combinations, it is best to have a compatible film-processing system.

Processing Steps

The four steps to be considered in film processing are developing, fixing, washing, and drying. The developer is an alkaline solution that converts exposed silver halide crystals to metallic silver by a chemical reaction. This reaction is often called a reduction process because the silver ion is said to be reduced to metallic silver.

The developer contains water, which is a solvent for the other chemicals and softens the film's emulsion. Hydroquinone is the main ingredient of developer solution with phenidone and Metol® as secondary agents. Hydroquinone and elon are combined for manual processing and hydroquinone and phenidone for rapid processing. These chemicals, when combined, have many electrons that are easily released to neutralize the positive silver ions in the film emulsion. Hydroquinone is responsible for bringing out the blackest shades on the radiograph, whereas phenidone influences the gray shades. Glutaraldehyde (hardener) is included in the developer for automatic processing. It is added to control emulsion swelling.

Unexposed silver halide crystals have a positive electrostatic charge whereas exposed silver halide crystals have a negative electrostatic charge. Because the electrostatic charge of the developer chemicals is negative, the chemicals cannot penetrate the silver halide crystal *except* in the region of exposure or where there are sensitized specks. In these areas, the developer chemicals penetrate through to the exposed specks and reduce the silver ions to atomic silver, Figures 9-13 and 9-14. Unexposed silver halide crystals are not changed or affected by the developer solution.

Figure 9-13. Development amplifies the latent image. Only crystals that contain a latent image are reduced to metallic silver by the addition of developer.

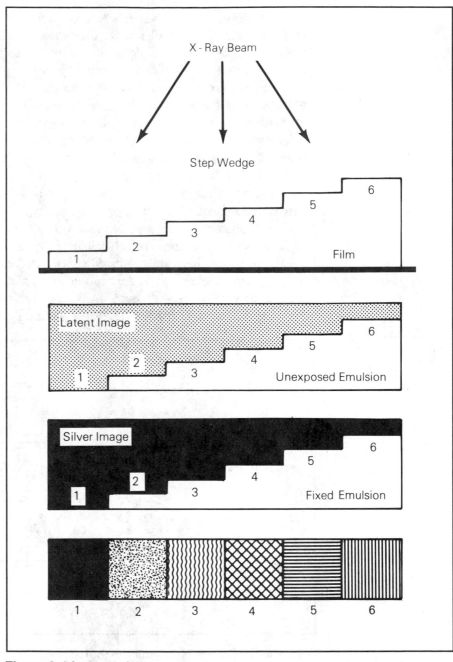

Figure 9-14. Latent image process

Other ingredients in the developer consist of an activator (such as sodium carbonate), a preservative, and restrainer. The preservative sodium sulfite serves to retard the activity of the reducing agents, thereby decreasing oxidation. Oxidation is undesirable because the chemicals' activity level declines when combined with oxygen. Potassium bromide, a restrainer, limits the action of the developer chemicals to the reduction of *only* the exposed silver halide crystals. Without proper balance provided by the restrainer, the unexposed silver halide crystals would be attacked. This ingredient is not required when mixing replenishment chemicals because bromide is reposited into the solution as each film is developed. Because the potassium bromide is used when mixing the initial developer solution, it is commonly called "starting solution" or "starter."

Replenishment of chemicals is very important in providing diagnostic-quality radiographs. Replenishment is used to restore both developer and fixer chemicals to their original strength. As films are processed, they retain a certain amount of chemicals and this depletes the solution level and the chemical strength. In automatic film processing, a pump replenishes the chemicals each time a film is processed; in manual film processing, the amount and rate of replenisher chemical must be performed by the radiographer. In manual processing, replenishment is usually done daily and is based upon the number and size of the films processed.

The fixer is an acidic solution that clears or removes unexposed silver halide crystals from the film emulsion. It also hardens and fixes the film so that it can be maintained as a permanent record. The fixer, like the developer, contains water as a solvent, which serves as a base for the other chemicals. Acetic acid allows the use of potassium alum as a hardening agent but also neutralizes any alkaline developer solution remaining on the film. The clearing agent ammonium thiosulfate (hypo) removes unexposed and undeveloped silver halide crystals from the emulsion. Hardening agents, either aluminum chloride or potassium alum, control the swelling of the emulsion and help to shrink it. Sodium sulfite is included as a chemical preservative to reduce oxidation.

A film must be properly washed to remove processing chemicals. In manual processing, films must be washed in continuous circulating fresh water. Automatic processors accomplish this by a constant inflow of water.

Automatic film processors have a system that produces a dry film. In the manual system, films may be either air dried on racks or placed in a film dryer. Films should be thoroughly dry before being filed and stored. Wet or damp radiographs may stick together, rendering them useless for future reference.

Manual-Processing Considerations

The maintenance of chemical strength, tank level, and temperature are the most important considerations in manual processing. The temperature of the chemicals is maintained by water circulating around the inner tanks and by the room temperature. In the manual method, processing time is closely related to temperature and chemical strength. Manufacturers usually recommend developing at 68° F for five minutes. Rapid manual-processing chemicals are available that allow development times of less than five minutes. Manual-processing tanks must be kept covered when not in use to prevent oxidation. Figure 9-15 illustrates the conventional arrangement of a small tank unit and Figure 9-16 a single wash compartment.

Conventional Arrangement of a Small Tank Unit (*Top View*):

    A. Master Tank
    B. Developer Tank
    C. Acid Rinse Bath, if Used
    D. Water Rinse or Washing Section
    E. First Fixing Tank
    F. Second Fixing Tank

Figure 9-15. Small tank unit *(top view)*

The steps in manual processing and a suggested time temperature chart, Figures 9-17 and 9-18, are provided by the Eastman Kodak Company. Exercise 9-8 in the appendix provides guidelines for manually processing film.

Automatic Film Processing

Automatic film processing, introduced in the late 1950s, has several advantages over manual processing. It is a clean and dry process; the operator does not have contact with the processing chemicals. Automatic processing is definitely faster. Some processors provide a finished film in as little as ninety seconds. The most important advantage is the constant control over chemical temperature and chemical strength. Chemicals used in automatic processing are more concentrated than in the manual process, and a higher temperature is used.

Figure 9-16. Single wash compartment

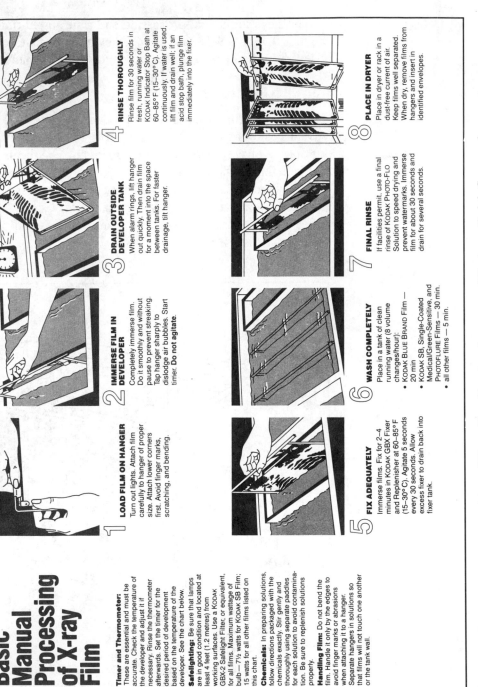

Basic Manual Processing of X-ray Film

Timer and Thermometer: These are essential and must be accurate. Check the temperature of the developer and adjust it if necessary. Rinse the thermometer afterwards. Set the timer for the desired period of development based on the temperature of the developer. See the chart below.

Safelighting: Be sure that lamps are in good condition and located at least 4 feet (1.2 metres) from working surfaces. Use a KODAK GBX-2 Safelight Filter, or equivalent, for all films. Maximum wattage of bulb—7½ watts for KODAK SB Film; 15 watts for all other films listed on this chart.

Chemicals: In preparing solutions, follow directions packaged with the chemicals exactly. Stir gently and thoroughly using separate paddles for each solution to avoid contamination. Be sure to replenish solutions properly.

Handling Film: Do not bend the film. Handle it only by the edges to avoid finger marks or abrasions when attaching it to a hanger. Separate hangers in solutions so that films will not touch one another or the tank wall.

1 LOAD FILM ON HANGER
Turn out lights. Attach film carefully to hanger of proper size. Attach lower corners first. Avoid finger marks, scratching, and bending.

2 IMMERSE FILM IN DEVELOPER
Completely immerse film. Do it smoothly and without pause to prevent streaking. Tap hanger sharply to dislodge air bubbles. Start timer. **Do not agitate.**

3 DRAIN OUTSIDE DEVELOPER TANK
When alarm rings, lift hanger out quickly. Then drain film for a moment into the space between tanks. For faster drainage, tilt hanger.

4 RINSE THOROUGHLY
Rinse film for 30 seconds in fresh, running water or KODAK Indicator Stop Bath at 60–85° F (15–30° C). Agitate continuously. If water is used, lift film and drain well; if an acid stop bath, plunge film immediately into the fixer.

5 FIX ADEQUATELY
Immerse films. Fix for 2–4 minutes in KODAK GBX Fixer and Replenisher at 60–85° F (15–30° C). Agitate 5 seconds every 30 seconds. Allow excess fixer to drain back into fixer tank.

6 WASH COMPLETELY
Place in a tank of clean running water (8 volume changes/hour):
- KODAK BLUE BRAND Film — 20 min
- KODAK SB, Single-Coated Medical/Green-Sensitive, and PHOTOFLURE Films — 30 min.
- all other films — 5 min.

7 FINAL RINSE
If facilities permit, use a final rinse of KODAK PHOTO-FLO Solution to speed drying and prevent watermarks. Immerse film for about 30 seconds and drain for several seconds.

8 PLACE IN DRYER
Place in dryer or rack in a dust-free current of air. Keep films well separated. When dry, remove films from hangers and insert in identified envelopes.

Figure 9-17. Basic manual processing of X-ray film *(Reprinted courtesy of Eastman Kodak Company)*

KODAK Time-Temperature Processing Chart

FOR USE WITH: Kodak GBX Developer and Replenisher and Kodak GBX Fixer and Replenisher

	T-MAT	X-OMAT S, X-OMAT RP, X-OMAT L, Single-Coated Medical/Green-Sensitive	GPG, X-OMAT G, Ortho G, Ortho L, BLUE BRAND, X-OMAT Duplicating, Rapid Process Copy, X-OMAT AR	GPB, SB, X-MAT K, MIN-R, PHOTOFLURE	Ortho H
KODAK X-ray Films					
Develop — For time indicated below. **Do not agitate.** Check developer temperature before each use.					
68° F 20° C	8 Min	7 Min	5 Min	3½ Min	4 Min
72 22	7	6	4	3	3
76 24	5	4	3	2	2½
80 26.5	4	2½	2	1½	2
Rinse	For **30 seconds** in fresh, running water or KODAK Indicator Stop Bath at 60–85° F (15–30°C). **Agitate continuously.**				
Fix	Fix **2–4 minutes** in KODAK GBX Fixer and Replenisher. **Agitate 5 seconds in every 30 seconds.** KODAK RP X-OMAT Fixer and Replenisher or KODAK Rapid Fixer may be used.				
Wash	In clean, running water at 60–85° F (15–30°C) with approximately 8 volume changes per hour. Wash for **5 minutes except:** BLUE BRAND Film for 20 minutes; SB, Single-Coated Medical/Green-Sensitive, and PHOTOFLURE Films for 30 minutes.				
Dry	At room temperature in a dust-free area or a suitable drying cabinet. Temperature not to exceed 120° F (50°C).				

Replenishment instructions are different for each solution.
Follow the specific recommendations for the developer replenisher and fixer replenisher furnished with chemical concentrates.

Figure 9-18. Kodak time-temperature processing chart (*Reprinted courtesy of Eastman Kodak Company*)

Automatic processing systems include transport, water, recirculation, replenishment, and dryer systems. Each will be discussed briefly.

Transport System.   The transport system consisting of rollers, transport racks, and drive motors, moves the film through the chemical solutions. It also serves to continuously agitate the chemicals, which prevents settling of the solutions. The transport system begins at the feed tray located in the darkroom. As the film is gently pushed on the feed tray, rollers grip the edge and begin moving it through the processor, Figure 9-19. Microswitches located at the entry to the feed tray detect the film size and start the automatic chemical-replenishment pump. The rate at which the film is transported through the processing tanks is very carefully controlled by the roller system. Roller subassembly consists of one-inch-diameter transport rollers and three-inch master rollers. Most of the rollers, except for those at the feed tray entry, are located within a rack. This allows for easy removal to clean and service the assembly. The transport system is powered by a motor whose time is set to the manufacturer's specifications.

Figure 9-19. Crossover rack with ribbed guide shoes *(Reprinted courtesy of Eastman Kodak Company)*

Water System. The water system washes the film and helps to stabilize the temperature of the solutions. Incoming water into the processor is maintained by a thermostatic regulating device.

Recirculation System. The recirculation pump blends and mixes the developer and fixer solutions with replenishment solution. This is very important for maintaining the proper temperature and chemical-activity level of the solutions. Constant agitation keeps the solutions mixed and in contact with the film.

Replenishment System. Automatic-processing chemicals are replenished by replenishment pumps each time a film enters the feed tray rollers. Manufacturers recommend replenishment rates based on the number of films processed. This method assumes a common density to each film and bases the quantity of replenishment solution upon a known standard of silver halide conversion to metallic silver. Regular checks are required to assure that the replenishment rates are accurate. This process is considered part of a quality control program.

Dryer System. Automatic-processor drying consists of a blower system that disperses heated air around the film as it moves past.

Limited radiographers should be familiar with automatic-processing components. Each manufacturer provides detailed operating and maintenance manuals, and these should be consulted whenever questions arise. Also, most X-ray sales and service companies provide representatives who help answer technical film-processing questions.

Processing films in an automatic processor is a simple task. Exercise 9-9 in the appendix offers a step-by-step guide to automatic film processing.

Artifacts

Film artifacts are undesirable. They consist of a wide range of extraneous marks and areas of increased or decreased density (darkening) that interfere with the diagnostic value of the radiograph. Table 9-5 provides a list of common artifacts. They are caused by physical, mechanical, and chemical means and may be avoided if proper film handling and storage procedures and appropriate film-processing guidelines are observed. Table 9-6 provides a list of common problems and corrections related to handling and processing X-ray film. After films are processed they should be checked for artifacts. If artifacts are visible, the cause or source should be determined and corrected, Figures 9-20 through 9-23.

TABLE 9–5   ARTIFACTS AND SOURCES

ARTIFACT	SOURCE
Brown Stain	From old or oxidized developer (too much air has mixed with the solution)
Multicolored Stain	From poor rinsing
Yellowish Film	From exhausted or weakened fixer solution
Milky-white Film	From incomplete washing time
Streaking	From solutions that have not been stirred well or films not agitated well, films not rinsed adequately, poor circulation in automatic processor, withdrawing film after it had started through the entrance assembly of the processor. In manual processing, check the wire hanger clips for chemical residue. Clean with a stiff brush.
Crinkle Marks	From kinking the film during handling
Reticulation	Are weblike marks that appear in the emulsion when there are extreme differences in the processing solutions. Refer to appendix for illustration.
Hesitation Marks	From automatic processor when the film hesitates or stops and there are increased density lines across the film. Refer to appendix for illustration.
Guide Shoe Marks	From automatic processor when film guide racks are not lined up properly with the rollers closest to them. Refer to appendix for illustration.

Figure 9-20. Both images on this radiograph were caused by mishandling the film. The single arrow demonstrates a *crinkle mark*, which can occur if the film is bent. The double arrows show an artifact caused by pressure on the surface of the film.

Figure 9-21. Kink, crinkle, or half-moon artifact caused by mishandling of the film. A white crinkle mark is caused by bending the film prior to exposure. A black crinkle mark is caused by bending the film after exposure and prior to processing.

Figure 9-22. Pressure artifact resulting from closing the drawer of the film bin on the sheet of film

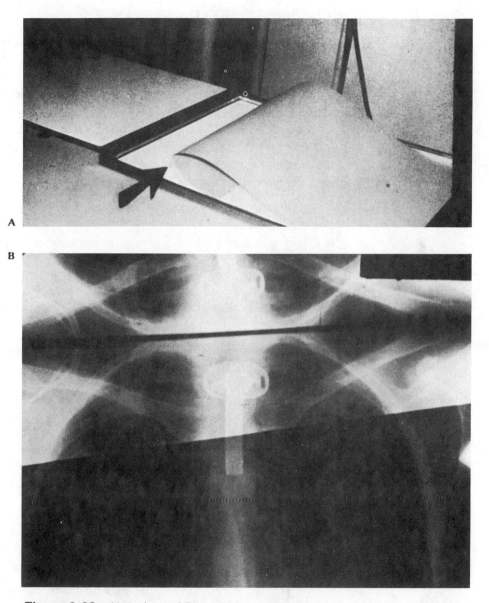

Figure 9-23. A) A sheet of film may be accidentally loaded into the cassette in a folded position; B) The artifact in this radiograph resulted from loading the film into the cassette in a folded position.

AUTOMATIC-PROCESSOR MAINTENANCE

Automatic processors, like any electromechanical equipment, must have regular service and repair. Processor maintenance consists of the usual daily, weekly, and monthly care as well as preventive and nonscheduled maintenance. Generally, limited radiographers are not expected to perform preventive or repair maintenance; such procedures are usually performed by skilled service people. Radiographers are, however, expected to perform the usual daily processor care, maintain a designated preventive maintenance schedule and records, and recognize the need for nonscheduled repair. Suggestions for daily processor care follow:

- Clean crossover rollers (use water and a nonabrasive, lint-free cloth), Figure 9-24.
- Observe all moving parts for wear. Report anything unusual to immediate supervisor.

Figure 9-24. This radiographer is removing and cleaning crossover rollers from an automatic processor as part of a daily maintenance routine.

- Check level of replenishment solutions in storage tanks.
- Drain the wash tank and offset the processor lid at night (this prevents the build up of algae in the tanks).

Preventive maintenance should be regularly scheduled. Each manufacturer will suggest a planned program that should be followed. Consult with company representatives or X-ray sales and service personnel to determine the best schedule to follow.

Nonscheduled maintenance is the most dreaded because it means a mechanical or electrical failure within the processor. The number of these incidents can be reduced with a regular preventive maintenance program. How does one know if something is wrong? Generally, automatic-processor problems will first become evident on the films. Unusual scratches, lines, marks, or improper processing of the films will be noticed. Also, some problems will be noticed first as an unusual operating sound. Limited radiographers are not expected to diagnose such problems, but before making a service call, it is important for the radiographer to note any detail noticed, e.g., nature of the problem, visual appearance of films processed, unusual sounds, or signs of leaks or mechanical failure. It is also a good idea to check all temperature and chemical controls before reporting the problem. Table 9-6 lists common film handling and processing problems and possible corrections.

SENSITOMETRY

Sensitometry is the study of how radiographic film responds to radiation exposure and processing conditions. Sensitometry is used to measure and predict how film density will change as radiation exposure factors and processing conditions change. By monitoring these responses, it provides early detection of equipment malfunctions before they can cause serious operational problems that may result in repeat of patient examinations. Changes in the film characteristics can be easily detected by sensitometry when radiation exposure and processing conditions are constant. Changes in processing conditions may also be identified when film-screen system and radiation exposure factors are constant. Sensitometry measurements include those visibility factors of density, contrast, and fog.

TABLE 9–6 HANDLING AND PROCESSING X-RAY FILM: COMMON PROBLEMS AND CORRECTIONS

PROBLEM	CAUSE	CORRECTION
Radiograph too dark	1. Overexposure 2. Overdevelopment 3. Concentrated replenishment	1. Reduce exposure 2. Adjust development time (manual). Check temperatures of water and solutions (automatic). 3. Adjust replenishment
Radiograph too light	1. Underexposure 2. Underdevelopment 3. Exhausted replenishment	1. Increase exposure 2. Adjust development time (manual). Check temperatures of water and solutions (automatic). 3. Adjust replenishment
Fog on radiograph	1. Chemical vapor exposure 2. Storage temperatures too high or humidity too high 3. Expiration date on film has passed 4. Safelight exposure 5. X-ray exposure 6. Pressure	1. Store film away from hydrogen sulfite, hydrogen peroxide, terpene, mercury 2. Store film in appropriate place, temperature 3. Regularly rotate film stock and use film before expiration date 4. Use recommended filter color, bulb wattage, and location of safelight from film-loading bench 5. Store film in appropriate place 6. Do not apply pressure or stack stored film boxes

TABLE 9–6 (CONT'D)

PROBLEM	CAUSE	CORRECTION
Black circular spots	Developer on film before development	Avoid developer splashes on film
White circular spots	Fixer on film before development	Avoid fixer splashes on film
Branched black marks	Static electricity discharge	Use proper film-handling procedures. Avoid clothing that contains excessive static build-up, such as nylon.
Crescent-shaped black marks	Bend in the film after exposure	Use proper film-handling procedures
Crescent-shaped white marks	Bend in the film before exposure	Use proper film-handling procedures
Yellow or brown stains	Exhausted developer; exhausted fixer	Replace solution

A characteristic curve, sometimes called H & D curve and first used in 1890 for photography analysis by Hurter and Duffield, is used to measure and predict film response to changes. The curve looks like a letter S when plotted on a graph, Figure 9-25. The graph is plotted by exposing a film and plotting the density levels against a logarithm of the various exposure levels.

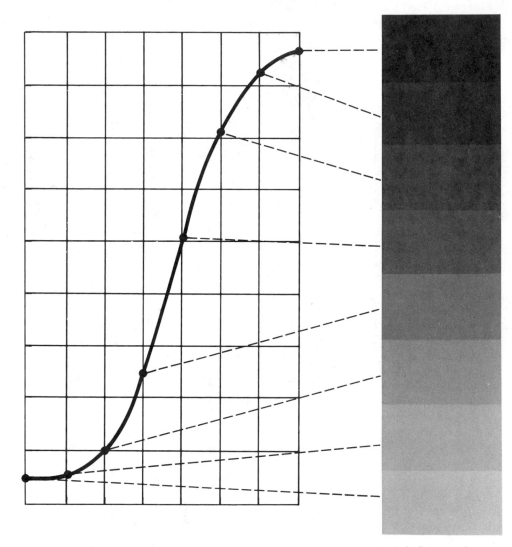

Figure 9-25. The H & D curve *(Reprinted courtesy of Eastman Kodak Company)*

Sensitometry Methods

There are three methods of performing sensitometry: step-wedge pentrometer and medium exposure, sensitometer exposure, and pre-exposed sensitometry strips. Most limited radiographers will be involved with only the third and easiest method of sensitometric measurement; thus, this is the only method that will be described.

In the procedure for pre-exposed sensitometry test strips, the strips are purchased and are stored in the film bin. When processed, the strips will have areas of increasing density. The processed strips are analyzed in a densitometer, an instrument with a light-sensing device. The amount of light transmitted through each segment on the strip is measured. A characteristic curve should result when this information is recorded and analyzed. Strips are regularly processed and the densities evaluated. This is a very common, widely used method today. Sensitometry application to film processing will be discussed in more detail with radiographic exposures.

SILVER RECOVERY

Silver, a treasured metal, can be recovered from fixer processing chemicals. Silver can also be reclaimed from scrap film and purged radiographic films. Why recover silver? Silver recovery is one way to salvage a scarce natural resource and also provides a small monetary return. The unexposed silver halide is dissolved in the fixer as the radiograph progresses through the film-processing cycle. There are two common methods used to recover silver from the fixer solution: metallic replacement and electrolytic recovery, Figure 9-26.

Metallic replacement removes silver from the used fixer solution by chemically replacing silver with another metal. As the metal dissolves, the silver moves to the bottom of the container and is removed.

Electrolytic recovery uses electrodes placed in the fixer tank. An electric current causes the silver to attach to one of the electrodes.

To determine which silver recovery system to use, consult with the processor manufacturer or an X-ray service company. Some X-ray service companies will perform routine processor maintenance and cleaning in return for the silver recovery profit.

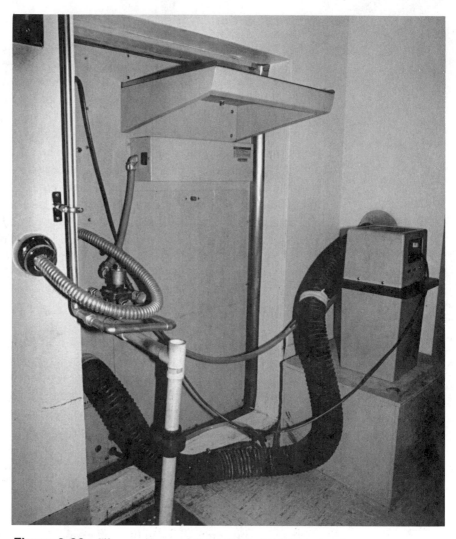

Figure 9-26. Silver-recovery system attached to an automatic processor

REVIEW QUESTIONS

1. What are the two main parts of radiographic film?
   a) emulsion and gelatin
   b) gelatin and silver halide crystals
   c) film base and gelatin
   d) film base and emulsion

2. A cassette or direct exposure film holder must be
   a) lighttight
   b) airtight and lightweight
   c) adhesive and airtight
   d) waterproof and fluorescent

3. To reduce excessive radiation exposure to the patient, the following combination should be used:
   a) screen film and cassette
   b) direct exposure film and cassette
   c) direct exposure film and cardboard holder
   d) screen film and cardboard holder

4. The active (phosphor) layer of an intensifying screen
   a) converts X-ray photons to visible light
   b) makes the screen lightproof
   c) decreases buildup of static electricity
   d) converts X-ray energy into light energy

5. Rare-earth intensifying screens have the following advantage compared to calcium-tungstate intensifying screens:
   a) provide more visible detail
   b) require less radiation and shorter exposure time
   c) permit shorter exposure time but require more radiation
   d) less costly

6. Select the spectral matching combination which would reduce the patient's radiation dose.
   a) high-speed film and high-speed screen
   b) high-speed film and low-speed screen
   c) low-speed film and high-speed screen
   d) low-speed film and low-speed screen

7. Radiographic film is *not* sensitive to
   a) chemicals
   b) heat
   c) pressure
   d) odors

8. Unexposed silver halide crystals are removed from the film in the _____ stage of film processing.
   a) development
   b) wash
   c) final rinse
   d) fixation

9. The following is *not* a component of the fixer:
   a) reducing agent
   b) preserver
   c) hardener
   d) acidifier

10. In an automatic processor, the chemicals are agitated by the _____ system.
    a) replenishment
    b) water
    c) roller
    d) dryer

11. If a radiograph is fogged, the radiographic density will
    a) increase
    b) decrease
    c) no change
    d) none of the above

12. Radiographic film is more easily fogged
    a) before being loaded into a film holder
    b) after its exposure to X rays but before processing
    c) after processing
    d) after storage

13. The processing solution with an acid ph is
    a) developer
    b) fixer
    c) rinse
    d) wash

14. Fogging of the radiograph produces increased
    a) density
    b) contrast
    c) distortion
    d) recorded detail

REFERENCES

1. *The Fundamentals of Radiography*, 12th ed, p. 34 Health Sciences Markets Division, Eastman Kodak Company, Rochester, New York 14650.
2. Ibid., p. _____.
3. Sweeney, Richard J., R.T., F.A.S.R.T., *Radiographic Artifacts: Their Cause and Control*. Philadelphia: J. B. Lippincott Company, 1983.

BIBLIOGRAPHY ▬▬▬▬▬▬▬▬▬▬▬▬▬▬▬▬▬▬▬▬▬▬

Bushong, Stewart. *Radiologic Science for Technologists, Physics, Biology, and Protection*. 3d ed. St. Louis: The C. V. Mosby Company, 1984.

Cullinan, Angeline, R. T. (R), F.A.S.R.T. *Producing Quality Radiographs*. Philadelphia: J. B. Lippincott Company, 1987.

Lamel, David A., Reynolds F. Brown, John W. Shaver, Eleanor Sirafinejad, Peter Weinberg, and Joseph S. Arcarese. *The Correlated Lecture Laboratory Series in Diagnostic Radiological Physics*. U. S. Department of Health and Human Services.

Morgan, James A. *The Art and Science of Medical Radiography*. 3d ed. The Catholic Hospital Association, 1971.

Quinn, B. Carroll. *Principles of Radiographic Exposure Processing and Quality Control*. 3d ed. Springfield, Illinois, Charles C Thomas, Publisher, 1985.

Selman, Joseph. *The Fundamentals of X-ray and Radium Physics*. 7th ed. Springfield, Illinois, Charles C Thomas, Publisher, 1985.

CHAPTER

10

Evaluation of Radiographic Quality: Image Evaluation

CHAPTER OUTLINE

Introduction
Image-Quality Considerations
Preparation of Image Production
Radiographic-Film Processing
Identification of Corrective Factors for Poor Radiographic Quality
    Radiographic-Image Evaluation

OBJECTIVES

Upon completion of the chapter, the student will demonstrate knowledge, facts, and principles presented through oral and written communication at a level deemed competent and will meet the task objectives by demonstrating the specific behavior as identified in the terminal performance objectives of the procedures.

1. Identify a minimum of four factors that control film quality.
2. List some actions that are generally acceptable when adjustments are required on radiographs that are too dark or too light.
3. Identify appropriate steps for proper radiographic positioning technique that affect film quality.
4. List five basic steps that relate to maintaining proper processing technique.
5. Identify and describe an appropriate method for critique of exposure factors for evaluation of radiographic quality.

TASKS (see Appendix):

1. Given example radiographs showing both acceptable and poor radiographic quality, evaluate the radiographs according to appropriate criteria.
2. Given radiographs showing processing factors used, identify the problem and list probable causes and corrective actions.

INTRODUCTION

Evaluation of radiographic quality is a process of visually assessing the image recorded on a film. When we look at a black and white photograph, we automatically look for detail in a person's face, a building, a landscape, and so forth. If the photograph is too dark, too light, or motion is seen, information is lost.

The radiographer must possess the appropriate knowledge and skills to visualize, inspect, and determine that technical qualities of the radiographic image are satisfactory. This chapter will address photographic qualities related to visual concepts of a recorded radiographic image. Visual inspection of the finished radiographic image under proper illumination (placed on a viewbox) will reveal most black-and-white (photographic) deficiencies related to too much or too little milliampere seconds (mAs), kilovoltage peak (kVp), or source-to-image distance receptor (SID).

Evaluation of the radiographic image includes multiple factors that are referred to in sum as *photographic effect* or *radiographic quality*. These factors have been dealt with fundamentally in chapter 8 under exposure factors mA, time, mAs, kVp, and SID. Relative to radiographic quality, these exposure factors may be discussed in terms of the following areas: 1) image-quality considerations, 2) preparation of image production, and 3) radiographic film processing.

IMAGE-QUALITY CONSIDERATIONS

Most people have difficulty seeing what they are not prepared to see. For example, in a stroll through a black-and-white photographic exhibit in a gallery or museum, many viewers react only in terms of whether they like or dislike the subject of a photograph. Others, who have had training in photography or art, additionally react to the shapes, lines, movement, contrast of light and dark, perspective, etc. Details and the quality of the overall effect, rather than the subject, are probably more important to the trained viewer.

In radiography, through educational preparation, the operator must learn about exposure factors and the often delicate balance and interaction between these factors in order to produce film images and then to evaluate the quality of those images. To assess a finished radiograph, the radiographer's preparation must include knowledge of the following "chain" of factors, their interplay, and their effects on the finished image: the exact mA, time, and kVp; patient's history and present condition; the centimeter measurement of the body part being examined; the processing time and temperature; and any variation in these factors that may have occurred before or during exposure of the image. Knowing these factors and their interactions is crucial when it becomes necessary to repeat a radiograph. The radiographer who produced the initial image should conduct the second attempt to avoid making the same errors or a different error.

PREPARATION OF IMAGE PRODUCTION

When preparing to produce a radiographic image, the operator should employ a systematic approach in order to avoid mistakes. Simple criteria in the form of a checklist should be followed. Because radiographic quality is affected by improper positioning, these criteria should include steps to avoid poor positioning, which often results in repeating radiographs. Such a checklist should include the following procedures:

1. Carefully read the request for radiographic examination to assure that you are very clear on the doctor's instructions regarding what radiographic procedure(s) has been ordered. If there is doubt, confirm the radiographic procedure with the doctor.

2. Identify the patient by *asking* his/her name. Do not suggest: "Are you Mr. Doc?" Rather, simply ask "What is your name, Sir?" If the patient cannot respond, check the arm band or follow the appropriate procedure according to office or departmental policy.

3. The patient must be placed appropriately, according to certain basic principles of radiographic positioning.

   a. Proper radiographic positioning may be effective only when applied with sound knowledge of human structure.

   b. Prior to examination, the patient must be given proper instructions regarding the radiographic procedure.

   c. The patient must be made comfortable to avoid the interactive pull of muscle strain that can result in motion.

   d. The patient's entire body must be positioned so that alignment is achieved with the part of the anatomy being examined, to avoid a rotated or twisted effect that may obscure structural information.

   e. After proper body position has been obtained, it is essential that the part being examined be immobilized. Effective mobilization devices that tend to reduce motion are sandbags, tape, or compression bands.

(Although the next three checklist items, f–h, do not all pertain to positioning, each step is crucial to production of an image as a whole.)

   f. Only a film size that adequately includes the anatomical part being examined is necessary. The part in focus is placed in the film's center and a small unexposed border around the image at the film's edges (½″ to 1½″) should be visible. The border indicates exposure limitation.

   g. A very important geometric factor is to place the long axis of the anatomical part being examined, parallel to, in the center of, and adjacent to the long axis of the film. This avoids magnification of the structure and/or distortion.

   h. The central ray must be directed perpendicular to the long axis of the film and to the center of the film so that it passes through the center point of the structure.

4. Identify the film with an appropriate marker (usually lead). Place the marker parallel with the long axis of the part being radiographed in the outer margins of the film, outside the structure.

5. Measure the part being examined and select the exposure factors—mAs, kVp, and SID (usually standardized, but check to make sure). Measure the part being examined and *set kVp* unless using automatic exposure.

6. Before making exposure, give the patient final instructions and make a final check of the patient's whole body position. Specifically check the part being radiographed to assure that the position has not changed.

7. While constantly observing the patient through a leaded window, observe the mAs reading on the control console for correct exposure. *Do not* hold your head outside the protection booth to talk to the patient during exposure.

8. Return the patient to the waiting area after completion of all films. It is not wise to leave an unstable patient unattended in the room.

9. Check the film after processing and if radiographic quality is visible, release patient.

Although initially it may seem that these criteria are burdensome, they may be applied in a few seconds once the operator becomes familiar with following all of the steps in a systematic manner.

RADIOGRAPHIC-FILM PROCESSING

You have already learned about what is involved in film processing in chapter 9. Because film processing, like radiographic image production, also involves a chain of events, it is necessary to observe that certain processing elements are constant at all times under any conditions:

1. The time and temperature of the processor must remain at constant levels. Any change in time of processing or degree of temperature will be quickly noticed in the image.

2. Processor water flow must be constant and maintained at adequate flow pressure.

3. All hoses to the automatic processor and its replenishment tanks must be open, not kinked or clogged, cutting off chemical flow.

4. The processor must have a schedule for regular maintenance and preventive maintenance.

5. Processor care is generally coordinated with a processor-maintenance person. Day-to-day care of the processor is the responsibility of the radiographer and any others who are involved in equipment care.

IDENTIFICATION OF CORRECTIVE FACTORS FOR POOR RADIOGRAPHIC QUALITY

Radiographic-Image Evaluation

There are three areas in which the sum of the radiographic image, in terms of photographic effect may be evaluated: 1) photographic factors, 2) geometric factors, and 3) accurate radiographic position.

The finished radiographic image will appear either correct or incorrect in the eye of the beholder. If the image is incorrect, then the operator must visually determine if the image is photographically deficient in contrast (kVp) or density (mAs), or if the processing is of poor quality.

When the completed radiograph has been placed on the illuminator (viewbox), the contrast and density (discussed in chapter 8) of the image should be such that all areas in the anatomy are visible. A rule of thumb is that if the image is so dark (black) that nothing is visible, the mAs should be cut back to one-fourth of what was originally used (e.g., reduce from 40 mAs to 10 mAs) and then determine whether or not the film is adequate for exposure. When the image is dark but some anatomy can be seen by using a bright light or spotlight, reduce the mAs by only one-half (e.g., from 40 mAs to 20 mAs).

Unless appropriate preparation for image production has taken place, i.e., the radiographer understands and has carefully selected mAs, kVp, and SID (usually standard), only guesses can be made—trial and error—to correct radiographic technique (density and contrast) of poor quality in a recorded image.

Except in the case of patient motion, geometric factors are seldom a problem because most are standardized. Errors involving blurring or distortion (shape, size) are generally related to improper positioning, incorrect body alignment, misjudgment of the patient size and shape (body habitus), or inexperience. When an image is assessed for quality, consideration should be given to the accuracy of all of the factors used to produce the image. Most often, when the image is of poor quality, overexposure or, less frequently, underexposure is the problem and is usually correctable by an adjustment of the exposure time. However, not all problems may be so simply corrected. Tables 10-1 and 10-2 provide some basic category information that may be useful for evaluating the quality of radiographic images.

Some problems are basic and relatively common in the production of radiographic images. By now you have probably determined that two of the most likely technique errors are too much density and poor positioning. Most technique and positioning errors generally occur because of the radiographer's lack of attention to details. Table 10-3 identifies a checklist that will acquaint the student with tasks that need to be applied each time a radiographic image is produced.

TABLE 10–1   RADIOGRAPHIC QUALITY CHART— IMAGE VISIBILITY

DENSITY: OVERALL IMAGE APPEARS OVEREXPOSED OR UNDEREXPOSED

Factors to be considered:

mAs: Review the amount of mAs used

kVp: Review measurement of the part for amount of kVp used (too much scatter)

Processing: Check processor temperature and time (rarely a problem)
Check for chemical contamination (fog)

(If the problem is not related to above areas, investigate further.)

CONTRAST: OVERALL IMAGE APPEARS FLAT AND GRAY OR ALL APPROPRIATE STRUCTURES ARE NOT PENETRATED

Factors to be considered:

kVp: Review the amount of kVp used and part measurement. A flat gray appearance is usually caused by scattered radiation from excessive kVp.

mAs: Review the amount of mAs used. A gray appearance (added density) may be the result of using too much mAs.

Processing: Check processor temperature. A gray appearance (added density) may also result from processing at a temperature too high.
Check for chemical contamination (fog).

TABLE 10–2   RADIOGRAPHIC QUALITY CHART— GEOMETRIC FACTORS

IMAGE BLURRING: IMAGE APPEARS BLURRED ON THE FILM

Factors to be considered:

Patient breathed/moved:
Determine if patient breathed or moved during exposure. If the patient breathed, check the reason and use a faster time, if necessary, to eliminate motion. The most effective recourse against motion is a faster time. Immobilization with restraints and sandbag support should also be considered when motion is a problem.

Film-screen contact:
Although poor screen contact is rare today with the excellent construction of cassettes, it still occurs. When it occurs, the screens must be replaced in the cassette. It is unusual for screen contact to be a problem with cassette sizes other than $14'' \times 17''$.

DISTORTION: SHAPE/SIZE OF IMAGE APPEARS DISTORTED

Factors to be considered:

SID/OFD:
If the part is or must be placed away from the film surface, the SID should be increased to reduce magnification of size caused by the increase in part-film distance. The part should be no more than $1\frac{1}{2}''$–$2''$ away from the film at $40''$ SID or $2\frac{1}{2}''$–$3''$ away from the film at $60''$ SID.

Tube angulation:
Elongation or foreshortening of the part is usually caused by incorrect alignment of the tube or part. Remember, the part to be examined must be parallel to the plane of the film and the tube directed perpendicularly (no angle) through the center point of the anatomy to be viewed. Whenever possible, it is more desirable to rotate the part and keep the anatomy parallel to the film than to angle the tube through the part.

POSITIONING: THE IMAGE APPEARS TO BE INCORRECTLY POSITIONED

Factors to be considered:

Relationship of anatomy to the film plane and relationship of the CR (central ray) to the anatomy:
Review exactly how the patient was aligned for proper position and how the part to be examined was aligned with the film plane. Poor positioning is a common error and is usually the result of working hurriedly or not checking the position carefully enough. Remember, only one patient can be done at any given time, so there is no need to rush and make mistakes.

TABLE 10–3   CHECKLIST FOR EVALUATING RADIOGRAPHIC QUALITY

Student's Name_____

Exposure Factors: mAs (mA/T)_____ kVp_____

Processing: Time_____ Temperature_____

Radiographic Procedure(s) Requested:

EVALUATION CRITERIA	YES	NO	CORRECTIVE ACTION
Anatomy centered on film			
All necessary anatomical borders are visible			
Right/Left/Date marker visible			
Adequate density (mAs)			
Adequate contrast (kVp)			
Magnification/distortion visible			
Adequate detail/definition visible			
Gonad shielding visible (if req.)			
Collimation (clear border edge)			
Artifacts/visible			
Appropriate film direction placement			

REVIEW QUESTIONS

1. To evaluate radiographic quality means to
   a) visually assess a recorded image
   b) visually inspect a finished radiograph
   c) visualize, inspect, and determine correct image technique
   d) all of the above

2. The limited radiographer's educational preparation must include knowledge of
   a) mA, time, kVp, SID
   b) patient's history and condition assessment
   c) film processing
   d) all of the above

3. In the preparation of image production, which of the following must be done first?
   a) check room availability
   b) check with doctor
   c) carefully read examination request
   d) identify the patient

4. If an overall image appears overexposed or underexposed, generally the first factor to be considered for corrective action is
   a) kVp
   b) mAs
   c) mA
   d) processing

5. If an image has a flat or gray appearance, the problem most likely will be related to
   a) kVp
   b) mAs
   c) processing
   d) time

6. When all anatomy related to a particular image is not visually penetrated, the problem is most likely
   a) kVp too low
   b) kVp too high
   c) mAs too high
   d) mAs too low

7. A blurred image is most likely the result of
   a) motion
   b) kVp too low
   c) mAs too low
   d) no immobilization

8. The most common problem related to image size or shape is
   a) incorrect SID
   b) incorrect kVp
   c) incorrect positioning
   d) incorrect CR

9. If the image appears too long or too short, the _____ is probably not perpendicular to the structure.
   a) film plane
   b) CR
   c) tabletop surface
   d) tube

10. A slight change in the _____ will be seen on the image results almost immediately when film quality is evaluated.
    a) processor water flow
    b) processor time or temperature
    c) processor replenishment rates
    d) processor preventive maintenance

CHAPTER

11

Radiation Biology

CHAPTER OUTLINE

OBJECTIVES

Upon completion of the chapter, the student will demonstrate knowledge of facts and principles presented through oral and written evaluation.

1. Define common radiation terminology.
   a) Identify two sources of naturally occurring background radiation and man-made radiation.
2. Explain the ionization process as it relates to potential biologic damage in humans.

3. Draw an illustration of an atom that has undergone ionization and label the following:
   a) electric charge of the atom before ionization
   b) electric charge of the atom after ionization
   c) ion
   d) ion pair
4. Differentiate between electromagnetic and particulate radiation.
5. Describe the changes that occur on the cellular level as a result of ionization.
6. Draw an illustration to show what occurs in the target or direct-hit theory and the indirect-hit theory.
7. Discuss how the following factors influence biologic damage: 1) type of radiation; 2) amount of radiation received; 3) dose rate; 4) whole body or specific body part exposure.
8. Compare and contrast short-term and long-term radiation induced biologic effects.
9. Compare and contrast somatic effects and genetic effects of radiation.
10. Recall three factors influencing biologic radiosensitivity.

INTRODUCTION

Radiation biology is a branch of the biological sciences concerned with the effects of ionizing radiation on living organisms. By ionizing radiation we mean the types of electromagnetic and particulate radiation discussed in chapter 5. These are summarized in Table 11-1.

TYPES OF IONIZING RADIATION

There are many forms and sources of radiation. Some types of radiation, such as light from an ordinary light bulb, usually do not adversely affect humans; others, such as X rays, may be harmful. X rays are a type of ionizing radiation. Ionizing radiation causes changes in some of the atoms it passes through, causing them to separate into electrically charged positive or negative particles called ions. This ability to ionize the atoms of cells can make ionizing radiation harmful to living organisms.

Understanding the process of ionization is the key to understanding the harmful biologic effects of ionizing radiation and to recognizing radiographers' responsibility in minimizing radiation exposure to patients and themselves.

TABLE 11–1   TYPES OF IONIZING RADIATION
PARTICULATE RADIATION Source: Originates from the disintegration of the nucleus of radioactive atoms. Particles travel through space as alpha or beta particles.
ELECTROMAGNETIC RADIATION Source: Gamma rays originate from the disintegration of the nucleus of radioactive atoms. X rays originate from an X-ray tube production. Gamma rays and X rays travel through space at the speed of light, and have no mass or charge.

Humans have always been exposed to environmental or naturally occurring background radiation, Table 11-2. Background radiation comes from the sun, stars, and from naturally occurring radioactive materials in the soil and water. The actual amount of background radiation varies with the geographic area, its soil and rock composition, and its elevation above sea level, Figure 11-1. Humans receive more radiation exposure at high elevations because there is less atmospheric filtering of the radiation from outer space called cosmic rays. For example, an individual living in Denver, Colorado will receive twice the environmental cosmic radiation as an individual living at sea level.

A second major source of environmental radiation comes from naturally occurring radioactive materials, such as uranium, present in the ground, water, and air.

The amount of radiation exposure an individual receives depends on four factors: type of radiation, amount of radiation received, length of time exposed, and the specific parts of the body exposed. These are the underlying bases for radiation-protection measures and will be a basis for risk factors discussed in this chapter and radiation-protection procedures discussed in chapter 12.

TABLE 11–2 ANNUAL SOURCES OF U.S. POPULATION IONIZING-RADIATION EXPOSURE	
SOURCE	DOSE IN mSv (mrem)
Natural Sources	3.0 (300)
Radon	2.0 (200)
Other	1.0 (100)
Cosmic	0.28 (28)
Terrestrial	0.28 (28)
In the Body	0.39 (39)
Occupational	0.009 (0.9)
Nuclear Fuel Cycle	0.0005 (0.05)
Consumer Products	0.09 (9)
Miscellaneous Environmental	0.0006 (0.06)
Medical	0.5 (50)
Diagnostic X Rays	0.39 (39)
Nuclear Medicine	0.014 (14)
Total	3.6 (360)

ARTIFICIAL SOURCES OF RADIATION

Since the 1890s, when Roentgen discovered X rays, scientists have been experimenting with ionizing radiation. Much of the knowledge about the harmful effects of radiation has been gathered as a result of the human health consequences from various uses. From the early application of ionizing radiation for diagnostic imaging and treatment of disease to the use of radium for luminous watch dials, the effects and consequences have led to our current focus on exposure reduction and discrimination in applications. Today, radiation sources may be found in nuclear power plants, atomic weapons, ionization-type smoke detectors, airport luggage screening, and in many industrial and commercial applications. The annual dose of radiation received by humans from medical radiation exposure is estimated to be 93 millirems (see Table 11-2), whereas exposure from environmental sources is estimated to be approximately 108 millirems per year.

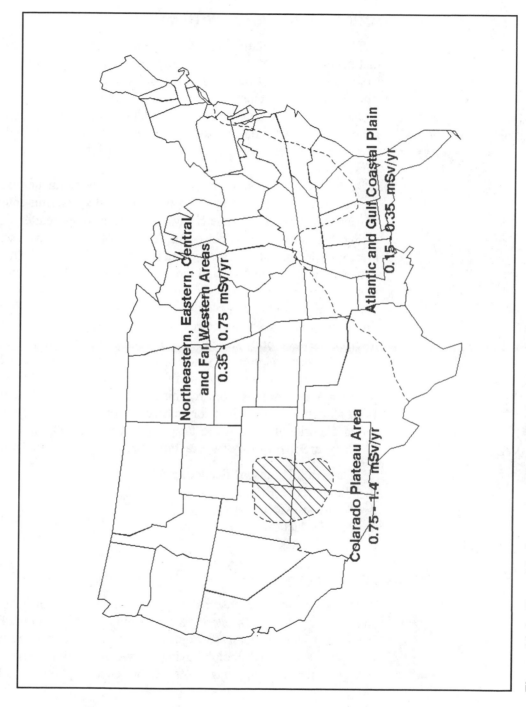

Northeastern, Eastern, Central
and Far Western Areas
0.35 - 0.75 mSv/yr

Atlantic and Gulf Coastal Plain
0.15 - 0.35 mSv/yr

Colarado Plateau Area
0.75 - 1.4 mSv/yr

Figure 11-1. Natural background radiation variation in the United States

INTERACTION OF RADIATION WITH MATTER

The effects of radiation on living organisms are a result of the ionizations that occur at the atomic level. During ionization, an electron(s) is removed from its energy shell resulting in a positively charged atom. The free electron can deposit its energy to surrounding tissue. As a result of ionizations, molecules may be altered to cause cellular damage that may result in abnormal cell function or loss of cell function. If enough cells have been damaged, the entire organ or organism may display symptoms of radiation damage.

A diagnostic X-ray beam passing through living matter will result in ionization in the cells comprising the matter. Because this interaction and ionization are random, some X rays will pass through matter without interacting. When interaction does occur, X-ray photons will give up their energy to atoms during the interaction, thus altering the atom. The interaction between the X-ray photons and the living matter resulting in energy transfer is called absorption or absorbed dose. The greater the absorbed dose, the greater the possibility of biologic effect. Because there is differential absorption of X rays in body structures of different densities, X rays can be used to visualize these body structures. For example, X rays are absorbed preferentially in bone as compared to soft tissue, thus producing the traditional radiographic image. Attenuation of the X-ray beam refers to any process that prevents X-ray photons from reaching the patient or the radiographic film. Both absorption and scatter, or redirection of an X-ray photon after it has interacted with an object, are factors affecting attenuation.

There are five types of interactions between X rays and matter:

1. Classical (Thomson) Scattering
2. Photoelectric Effect
3. Compton Effect
4. Pair Production
5. Photodisintegration

Classical Scattering

Classical scattering, also called Thomson scattering or coherent scattering, occurs when a low-energy X-ray interacts with an atom, Figure 11-2. The target atom becomes energized or "excited" and releases this extra energy as a scattered photon having a wavelength and energy equal to the energy of the original X-ray photon. This released photon is different from

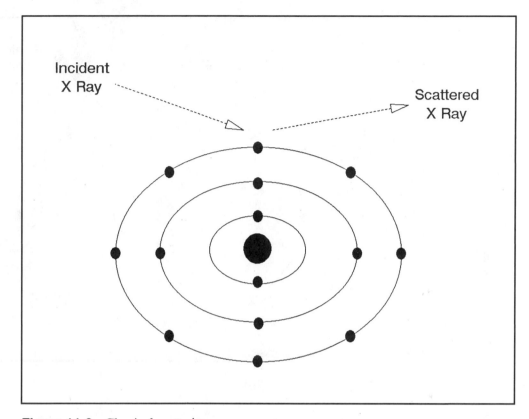

Figure 11-2. Classical scattering

the direction of the original X-ray photon; thus it is scattered. In this form of scattering, no energy transfer occurs, and therefore no ionization occurs. Classical scattering generally occurs in low kVp ranges; however, some occurs throughout the diagnostic kVp range, and is responsible for some small amount of radiographic-film fog.

Photoelectric Effect

The photoelectric effect or interaction occurs when the incident X-ray photon gives up all of its energy to an inner shell electron, Figure 11-3. When this occurs, an electron, called the photoelectron, is ejected from the atom, usually from the inner K or L shell, leaving a vacancy or "hole" to

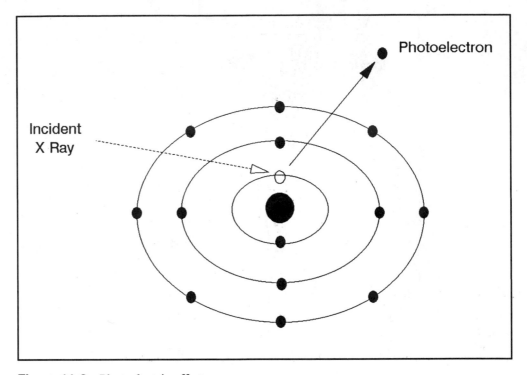

Figure 11-3. Photoelectric effect

be filled in the shell. When an inner-shell electron is removed from an atom, the resulting vacancy is filled by an electron from an outer shell. When an outer-shell electron fills an inner-shell vacancy, an X-ray photon may be emitted from the atom. This type of X ray is called characteristic radiation. Therefore, two types of secondary radiation result from a photoelectric interaction: characteristic X rays and photoelectrons.

Compton Effect

Compton scattering, first described in 1922 by physicist A. H. Compton, is the most common type of X-ray interaction in diagnostic radiology and is responsible for most scattered radiation. Compton scattering occurs when an X-ray photon interacts with an electron in the outer orbital shell of an atom. The outer-shell electron, called a Compton electron, is ejected from the atom and results in ionization of the atom, Figure 11-4. As a result of the interaction, the X-ray photon is redirected, with decreased energy and

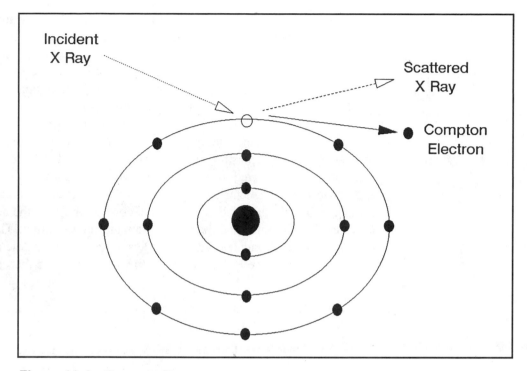

Figure 11-4. Compton effect

a longer wavelength. The scattered X-ray photon and the Compton electron have the energy to cause additional ionizing interactions with other atoms. Because Compton-scattered X-ray photons may be deflected in any direction, they are of especial concern in radiation protection. Those scattering back in the direction of the incident X ray are referred to as backscatter radiation.

Compton scatter radiation, like most scattered radiation, does not contribute to the diagnostic image. Rather, it causes radiographic-film fog and requires the use of lead shielding for protection of the radiation operator and patient.

CELL ANATOMY

The cell is the basic component of all living organisms. Each cell is a single functioning unit, capable of performing the processes essential for life. A single cell reacts to stimuli, ingests and metabolizes nutrients, synthesizes new materials, excretes wastes, and reproduces. Cells are involved in an ongoing process of obtaining and converting energy; and whatever threatens a cell's existence, in essence, poses a threat to the entire organism.

Collections of cells form tissue and tissues form organs. Organs with similar functions are called systems, Figure 11-5.

The cell has three basic parts: membrane, cytoplasm, and nucleus. The cell membrane is permeable, that is, it allows substances to pass into and out of the cell. The cytoplasm is a watery substance inside the cell. It contains many structures referred to as organelles, whose functions include receiving and converting raw materials into energy. The nucleus, separated from the cytoplasm by a double-walled membrane, consists of fluid (the nucleoplasm) in which the nucleolus and the chromatin material are found. The nucleolus is composed of ribonucleic acid (RNA), and deoxyribonucleic acid (DNA) in the chromatin. The RNA and DNA direct the activities that maintain cell

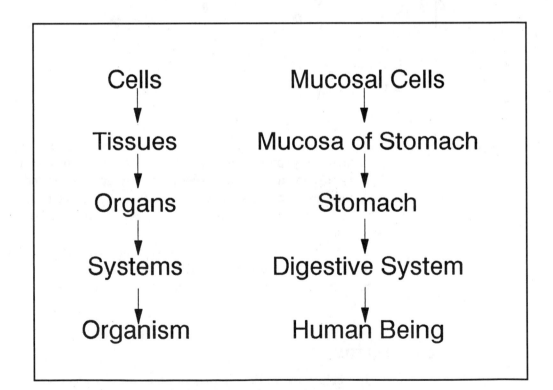

Figure 11-5. The organizational structure of a biological organism

life. Chromosomes that transmit the genetic code of hereditary information are composed of DNA. DNA is a complex molecule that is the carrier of the genetic code of the organism.

Cell division or multiplication is controlled by the nucleus. Two types of cell division occur: mitosis and meiosis. Genetic cells, such as spermatogonium, undergo meiosis; all other cells in the human body undergo mitosis.

In mitosis, the cell divides to form two cells. Mitosis occurs in five phases: interphase, prophase, metaphase, anaphase, and telophase.

Meiosis, or reduction division, differs from mitosis in that during cell division, the two identical cells produced each contain only one-half of the usual forty-six chromosomes.

Four things may happen when radiation strikes a cell: 1) it may pass through without damage to the cell; 2) it may damage the cell but the cell partially repairs the damage; 3) it may damage the cell so that the cell fails to repair itself but reproduces in damaged form; and 4) it may kill the cell.

RADIOSENSITIVITY

The so-called Law of Bergonié and Tribondeau attempts to explain the basis of living tissue radiosensitivity. The law states the following:

1. Immature, nonspecialized cells are most radiosensitive. Mature, specialized cells are most radioresistant.
2. Cells with a high metabolic level are radiosensitive.
3. Cells that are rapidly growing and dividing are radiosensitive.
4. Immature tissues and organs are radiosensitive.

Several physical factors should be considered in the determination of radiosensitivity: 1) linear energy transfer, 2) relative biologic effectiveness, 3) dose fractionation and protraction, and 4) individual biologic factors.

Linear Energy Transfer (LET)

LET is a unit of measure of the amount of energy transferred from radiation to tissue as a function of the distance the radiation travels in the tissue. The amount of energy transferred determines the amount of ionization, and thus, the potential biologic damage. As the LET of a radiation increases, the potential threat of biologic damage increases.

Relative Biologic Effectiveness (RBE)

RBE is a measure of the biological damage done by different types of ionizing radiation. For example, alpha particles are more damaging to the biological tissue than are X rays and thus have a higher RBE.

Dose-Response Relationship

A dose-response relationship refers to a point or level of exposure (dose) at which a response or reaction first occurs, Figure 11-6. The relationship between radiation and some biologic responses is a linear, non-threshold relationship. This means that any amount of ionizing radiation, no matter how small, may cause a biologic effect (response). The linear, non-threshold relationship model indicates that there is no amount of radiation exposure that is safe. It is assumed that all ionizing-radiation exposure presents the potential to cause biologic effect. Therefore, any such exposure requires the consistent use and application of radiation-protection measures to protect the patient and those performing the examination.

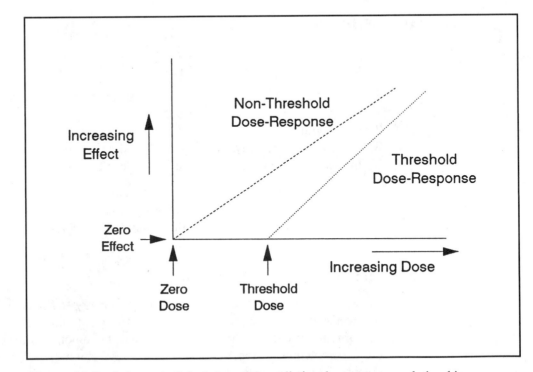

Figure 11-6. A theoretical depiction of the radiation dose-response relationship

Biologic Factors of Radiosensitivity

Several biological variables must also be considered when discussing cell radiosensitivity. These variables are based on the biological variations of individual organisms.

Age. Radiosensitivity is highest before birth and until maturity. Use of radiation-protection measures are very important for protection of the developing embryo and fetus, all children, and women who may have a likelihood of reproducing.

Sex. Scientific research indicates that females are approximately 5–10 percent more radiation-resistant than males.

Oxygen Effect. Oxygen enhances the effect of ionizing radiation on living organisms by increasing cell sensitivity.

Individual Variation In Response. Human cells are capable of recovering from radiation damage. The repair mechanism is dependent upon many biological and environmental factors.

There are two means of damaging a cell by radiation. These are the direct effect and the indirect effect. The direct effect refers to radiation interaction in which a photon directly interacts with a "target" or critical DNA molecule. In the indirect effect, a photon strikes a noncritical molecule, usually water, but the noncritical molecule transfers the ionization energy to the critical DNA molecule—an indirect effect. Because the human body is composed of approximately 80 percent water, it is believed that the greatest percentage of ionizations will occur as interactions between photons and water molecules. When a water molecule is ionized, it separates into free radicals. Free radicals are very chemically reactive forms of ions. The free radicals resulting from the radiolysis, or the breakdown of the molecule, have the potential to recombine to form a new water molecule or to combine with other radicals to form new molecules. It is believed that most of the effects of radiation on living organisms are a result of radiolysis or the indirect action caused when a photon interacts with a noncritical molecule, Figure 11-7.

The concept of a sensitive target or key molecule is called the target theory. The target theory states that there is a certain critical target molecule in a cell that must be inactivated in order to damage or kill the cell. Scientists believe that the DNA of a cell represents this target and is the area of the cell vital to cell life and replication.

Biologic effects may be classified as either short-term effects or long-term effects. Biologic effects from radiation fit into one or the other classification

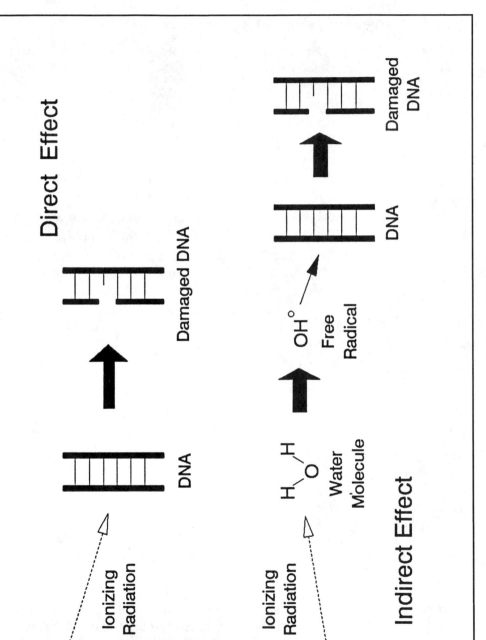

Figure 11-7. The direct and indirect effects of ionizing radiation on DNA

depending upon the length of time it takes for the effect to become evident or demonstrable. As previously discussed, several factors—such as type of radiation, amount of absorbed dose, and body area receiving the exposure—determine the type and intensity of the effect.

Short-term or early effects of exposure to radiation have classically been determined from studies of uranium miners, radium dial painters, survivors of the atomic bombs detonated in Japan during World War II, and survivors of nuclear power plant and nuclear industry accidents.

Short-term effects are found in the acute radiation syndrome, which includes but is not limited to gonadal dysfunctions, epilation (hair loss), depression of the white blood cells, and even death. Clinical signs and symptoms of short-term effects include nausea, vomiting, diarrhea, anemia, leukopenia, hemorrhage, fever, infection, and shock.

Long-term or late effects of radiation may result from small doses of radiation received over a number of years. Long-term effects may also be demonstrated in individuals who have been exposed to a single dose of radiation and have been in a latent period. Examples of long-term effects that have been demonstrated through epidemiologic studies of survivors of radiation exposures include the following:

■ *Local tissue effects.* An example of this effect is when the skin undergoes changes in its texture, elasticity, and appearance. It appears dry, chapped, and prematurely aged. Exposed skin may also exhibit an increase in skin lesions, both benign and malignant. These changes are both dose- and time-related.

■ *Chromosomal changes.* Chromosome damage may be exhibited as abnormal pairings, translocation, and other phenomena that can result in cell damage and dysfunction.

■ *Cataracts.* Radiation-induced cataracts were reported as early as the 1940s. The radiosensitivity of the lens of the eye has been demonstrated to be age-dependent. This means that the older the individual, the more susceptible one is to radiation-induced cataracts.

■ *Life span shortening.* It is suggested that, as a result of chromosomal mutations, the fitness and life span of an individual acutely exposed will be compromised and/or shortened. For this reason, the amount of radiation delivered in radiographic procedures should always be as low as reasonably possible to obtain the necessary diagnostic information, and radiation-protection measures should always be used.

Somatic and Genetic Effects.   The effects of radiation on living organisms are further classified as somatic or genetic. Somatic effects occur to the individual who has been exposed to ionizing radiation, whereas the genetic effects may not be apparent in the exposed individual but passed on to future generations through genetically damaged chromosomes.

Radiation Units of Measurement

One of the first units of measurement used for radiation was called the roentgen, after Professor Wilhelm Conrad Roentgen. A roentgen is the unit of measurement of the ionization of air by X rays or gamma rays. The ionizing potential of X rays is now measured in SI units as one coulomb/kilogram of air.

The units gray (Gy) and sievert (Sv) are used in measuring the effects of radiation on living organisms or materials. The gray expresses the energy per kilogram absorbed as a result of exposure to any type of radiation. One gray is that quantity of radiation that imparts one joule of energy to one kilogram. The gray replaces the rad (*r*adiation *a*bsorbed *d*ose), which was the absorption of one erg of energy by one gram of tissue.

The sievert is the unit used to express the quantity of radiation received in an occupational exposure. The gray expresses the quantity of absorbed dose and is an important indicator when considering biologic effects resulting from radiation exposure. But the sievert takes into account the type or source of the radiation and its potential for biologic damage. The sievert has replaced the rem (*r*ad or roentgen *e*quivalent *m*an).

The becquerel (Bq) is the unit used to measure radioactivity. A becquerel is a measure of the number of atoms disintegrating (decaying) per second in radioactive material. One becquerel is one radioactive disintegration per second. The becquerel replaces the old unit known as the curie.

SUMMARY OF HUMAN EXPOSURE TO IONIZING RADIATION

1. Biologic effects are dose-dependent (the greater the amount, the greater the effect).
2. Effects of a given exposure vary from person to person. Predicting exactly how an individual will respond is nearly impossible except at lethal-dose levels.

3. A great amount of radiation delivered over seconds, minutes, or hours is called an acute radiation exposure. Acute doses to the whole body are more dangerous than acute exposure to a specific body part.
4. There is controversy about the long-term effects of low doses of radiation; however, chronic low doses of radiation have been associated with a higher incidence of cancer.

REVIEW QUESTIONS

1. Organs with similar functions are called
   a) cells
   b) tissues
   c) organisms
   d) systems
2. Sources of radiation are
   1) man-made
   2) terrestrial
   3) cosmic
      a) 1 and 2
      b) 1 and 3
      c) 2 and 3
      d) 1, 2, and 3
3. In the photoelectric effect, the incident X ray interacts with a(n)
      a) inner-shell electron
      b) proton
      c) nuclear force field
      d) outer-shell electron
4. In the photoelectric effect, the incident X ray
   a) is completely absorbed
   b) is scattered at a lower energy
   c) is scattered at a longer wavelength
   d) is scattered at a higher frequency
5. A cell's sensitivity to radiation is determined by
   1) its degree of specialization
   2) how fast it grows
   3) its state of maturity

    a) 1 and 2
    b) 1 and 3
    c) 2 and 3
    d) 1, 2, and 3

6. Some long-term effects of radiation exposure are
   1) cataracts
   2) life span shortening
   3) epilation
    a) 1 and 2
    b) 1 and 3
    c) 2 and 3
    d) 1, 2, and 3

7. The radiation unit expressed as 1 J/kg is the
   a) roentgen
   b) rad
   c) gray
   d) rem

8. The units of dose that are equivalent are the
   a) rem and rad
   b) roentgen and rem
   c) gray and rem
   d) rem and sievert

9. A unit of radiation exposure is the
   a) rad
   b) roentgen
   c) gray
   d) rem

10. The units of radiation absorbed dose are the
   a) rad and roentgen
   b) roentgen and gray
   c) roentgen and sievert
   d) rad and gray

CHAPTER

12

Radiation Protection

CHAPTER OUTLINE

Introduction
Effective Dose Equivalent
Radiation-Protection Procedures
  The Patient
  Primary Beam Limitation
Pregnant Patient
Radiation-Protection Procedures for the Operator
  Cardinal Principles
  Protective Apparel
  The Pregnant Radiographer
Radiation Detection and Monitoring
  Personnel Monitoring Devices
  Survey Instruments for Area Monitoring

OBJECTIVES

Upon completion of the chapter, the student will demonstrate knowledge of facts and principles presented through oral and written evaluation and will meet the task objectives by demonstrating the specific behavior as identified in the terminal performance objectives of the procedures.

1. Identify the person who is responsible for evaluating each patient by considering the benefit-versus-risk principle prior to requesting a radiographic examination.
2. Define the term effective dose equivalent and state the annual occupational and nonoccupational MPD.

3. Explain the ALARA concept and give a minimum of two radiation-protection procedures supportive of the ALARA concept.
4. Summarize the main intent of the 1981 Consumer-Patient Radiation and Safety Act.

INTRODUCTION

The use of X-ray examinations to aid in the diagnosis of disease and injury is often considered to be a standard part of the diagnostic evaluation process. Yet few people realize that the physician must consider several factors before requesting a radiographic examination.

Each time a radiographic examination is indicated, the licensed medical practitioner must consider the potential diagnostic benefits to be gained from the radiographic examination versus the potential biologic harm to the patient resulting from radiation exposure. This decision is often called the benefit-versus-risk principle and must be considered each time a radiologic examination is requested. Once the decision to perform a radiographic procedure has been made by the doctor, it is the radiographer's responsibility to perform the examination and to follow all recognized radiation-protection guidelines. These guidelines consist of cardinal principles and procedures intended to reduce unnecessary radiation exposure to the patient and radiation operator. The main goal of all radiation-protection activities is to keep all radiation exposure *a*s *l*ow *a*s *r*easonably *a*chievable (ALARA). This chapter introduces current radiation-protection philosophy, the ALARA concept, effective-dose-equivalent guidelines, and radiation-protection procedures for the patient and radiation operator.

EFFECTIVE DOSE EQUIVALENT

Guidelines limiting the amount of radiation received by the general public and those individuals who use radiation in their work (occupational dose) have been established by several international and governmental agencies, Table 12-1.

The agencies named in Table 12-1 determine effective-dose levels and make recommendations that the Nuclear Regulatory Commission (NRC), a national agency, has the responsibility to enforce. There are five regional NRC offices that serve various geographic areas of the United States. Regional NRC offices accept collect telephone calls from employees who wish to register concerns or complaints about conditions or matters within radiologic facilities.

Traditionally, radiation-exposure limits have been expressed as the maximum permissible dose (MPD) of radiation to which the radiation-occupation worker or the general public can be exposed. Over the years, as knowledge of the injurious effects of radiation has increased, the MPD has been decreased, Table 12-2.

However, the MPD is no longer used as the criterion of radiation exposure in radiation protection. In 1987, the NCRP issued new guidelines for limits on exposure to ionizing radiation based on the dose equivalent. The dose equivalent is the product of absorbed radiation dose and the quality factor of the radiation. The quality factor for X rays, gamma rays, beta particles, and electrons is one. The name for the unit of dose equivalent is the sievert (Sv). The dose equivalent is further defined as the effective dose equivalent for partial-body irradiation of specific organs or tissues and the whole-body. Chapter 11 contains a detailed description of the units used to measure ionizing radiation. For purposes of comparison, a single chest X ray exposes the *patient* to approximately 0.1 mSv (10 mrem).

The recommendations on dose equivalent levels for individuals are based on the general ALARA concept and the negligible individual risk level (NIRL). The NIRL is not a radiation-exposure limit but is the level of risk below which it is unnecessary to control exposure to radiation. However, it may be stated that the NIRL corresponds to an annual effective dose equivalent of 0.01 mSv (0.001 rem).

TABLE 12–1	GROUPS RESPONSIBLE FOR ESTABLISHING RADIATION MAXIMUM-PERMISSIBLE-DOSE GUIDELINES
(ICRP)	International Commission on Radiological Protection
(NAS-BEIR)	National Academy of Sciences Advisory Committee on the Biological Effects of Ionizing Radiation
(NCRP)	National Council on Radiation Protection and Measurement
(UNSCEAR)	United Nations Scientific Committee on the Effects of Atomic Radiation

TABLE 12–2 OVERVIEW OF DOSE TRENDS		
YEAR	**APPROXIMATE DAILY DOSE**	
1902	100 mSv	10 rem
1925	2.0 mSv	0.2 rem
1928	1.5 mSv	0.15 rem
1936	1.0 mSv	0.1 rem recommended by the United States Advisory Committee on X-Ray and Radium Protection
1959	0.2 mSv	0.02 rem recommended by the National Council on Radiation Protection and Measurements

Effective-dose-equivalent limits differ for radiation workers and the general population. They are further modified by reference to specific organ or tissue exposures and embryo-fetus exposures. For occupational exposures, the annual effective-dose-equivalent limit is 50 mSv (5 rem). The dose-equivalent limit for the lens of the eye, an especially radiosensitive tissue, is 150 mSv (15 rem). For all other tissues and organs, including bone marrow, breast, lung, gonads, skin, and extremities, the limit is 500 mSv (50 rem). These and other recommendations are summarized in Table 12-3.

The age of the radiation worker is also a factor in exposure limitations. Previously, no one under eighteen years of age was allowed to work with ionizing radiation. The NCRP has stated that for educational and training purposes radiation workers less than eighteen years old be limited to an annual effective dose equivalent of 1 mSv (0.1 rem). In addition to annual dose limitations, a cumulative or lifetime dose limitation must be observed. This limit is determined by the age of the radiation worker. The total allowable cumulative exposure is the age (in years) of the worker times 10 mSv (1 rem). For example, a thirty-year-old radiographer is allowed a cumulative exposure of 30 × 10 mSv or 300 mSv (30 rem).

Guidelines for exposure limitations for the general public are less than for radiation workers. The effective dose equivalent for continuous or fre-

TABLE 12-3 DOSE-LIMITING GUIDELINES

OCCUPATIONAL PERSONNEL	ANNUAL DOSE EQUIVALENT	
Effective-dose-equivalent limit	50 mSv	(5 rem)
Lens of eye	150 mSv	(15 rem)
All other organs, organ systems, tissue	500 mSv	(50 rem)
Cumulative exposure	10 mSv × age	(1 rem × age)
NONOCCUPATIONAL (GENERAL PUBLIC)	**ANNUAL DOSE EQUIVALENT**	
Continuous or frequent exposure	1 mSv	(0.1 rem)
Infrequent exposure	5 mSv	(0.5 rem)
Lens of eye, skin, and extremities	50 mSv	(5 rem)
EDUCATION AND TRAINING EXPOSURES	**ANNUAL DOSE EQUIVALENT**	
Effective-dose-equivalent limit	1 mSv	(0.1 rem)
Lens of eye, skin, and extremities	50 mSv	(5 rem)
EMBRYO-FETUS EXPOSURES		
Total dose-equivalent limit to term	5 mSv	(0.5 rem)
Dose-equivalent limit in a month	0.5 mSv	(0.05 rem)

quent exposures is 1 mSv (0.1 rem) and for infrequent exposure 5 mSv (0.5 rem).

Embryo-fetal exposures are also considered separately. The total dose-equivalent limit for the embryo-fetus is 5 mSv (0.5 rem) and the dose-equivalent level in a month is 0.5 mSv (0.05 rem).

RADIATION-PROTECTION PROCEDURES

The Patient

The main goal of any radiation-protection procedure is to reduce unnecessary radiation according to the ALARA concept. Reducing unnecessary or excessive radiation exposure is a responsibility shared by everyone involved with radiologic examinations including the doctor, radiation operator, and all support staff. There are four major areas that relate to reducing radiation exposure: patient preparation, primary beam limitation, gonadal shielding, and technical factors.

Patient Communication. The first place where radiation-protection guidelines may be applied is when the examination is requested by the attending physician. It is the attending doctor's responsibility to explain why the radiologic examination is necessary, to answer patient questions, and to respond to any concerns about the nature of the examination. Poor communication between the doctor and the patient, the doctor and the radiation operator, and/or the operator and the patient may result in a repeat examination or even in the wrong patient being radiographed. Communication then becomes an important factor in reducing unnecessary or excessive radiation exposure. Patients have the right to know about the examination; and if inadequately informed, they may have questions or fears regarding the nature, purpose, or even value of the examination. Patients who do not understand what is going to happen or what is expected may even be reluctant to cooperate.

What responsibility does the medical radiographer have in regard to explaining the radiographic examination to the patient? It is the radiographer's responsibility to give the patient clear, concise instructions and to communicate in such a way that patients understand what is expected of them in order to complete the examination. If at any time the patient refuses to undergo the examination, the radiation operator should seek supervisory assistance. The radiation operator should *never* insist that the patient submit to any procedure against his/her will.

One way to ensure that each patient is informed regarding his/her radiographic examination is to take adequate time to explain the procedure so that the patient understands. The radiation operator should always answer patient questions within ethical limitations, and if asked a question s/he cannot answer, the radiation operator should seek supervisory assistance. Remember, patients have the right to be completely informed about their medical care and to have their questions answered.

Patient Preparation. Radiation protection also extends to patient preparation. Many repeat examinations occur as a result of inadequate patient preparation. It is important to ask the patient to remove all radiopaque objects from the area to be radiographed, such as necklaces, zippers, hair pins, and even long, braided hair. Remember that a repeat examination results in a repeat or double-radiation exposure to the patient.

During patient preparation and initial introductions, it is also important to give instructions regarding breath and motion control.

If positioning or immobilization devices are to be used, explain to the patient why they are needed and how they will be used. Talk to the patient before, during, and after the examination and let the patient be of assistance whenever possible.

Careful attention to radiographic positioning also helps reduce the number of retake radiographs and thus reduces unnecessary radiation exposure. Radiographers should never attempt a radiographic procedure if they are uncertain as to the correct procedure. If in doubt or just inexperienced, the radiographer should *STOP* and *ASK FOR HELP*.

Primary Beam Limitation

Primary beam limitation means using a device such as an aperture diaphragm, cone, or collimator to limit the useful or primary radiation beam to the area of clinical interest, thereby decreasing the area of body tissue irradiated. This in turn reduces the amount of secondary scattered radiation and also limits unnecessary exposure to the nearby tissue. A beam restrictor, however, is only as effective as the operator who uses the device. Therefore, it is important that radiation operators understand the basic operation of each type of beam restrictor and the operator's role in using the device.

The aperture diaphragm is a simple beam limitation device consisting of a flat piece of lead with a hole in the middle, Figure 12-1. The size and shape of the hole determine the size and shape of the radiographic beam.

An aperture diaphragm is constructed so that it fits directly below the X-ray tube window. One disadvantage of an aperture diaphragm is that each is designed to be used with a specific film size at a given distance. Because of this feature, it is not easily adaptable to various film sizes or distances. The variable aperture diaphragm device overcomes this disadvantage because it has a variable opening that can be adjusted for use with various film sizes and source-to-image distances.

Other simple beam-limitation devices are the cone (a circular metal tube with a flared end) and the cylinder (a long tube having the same diameter at

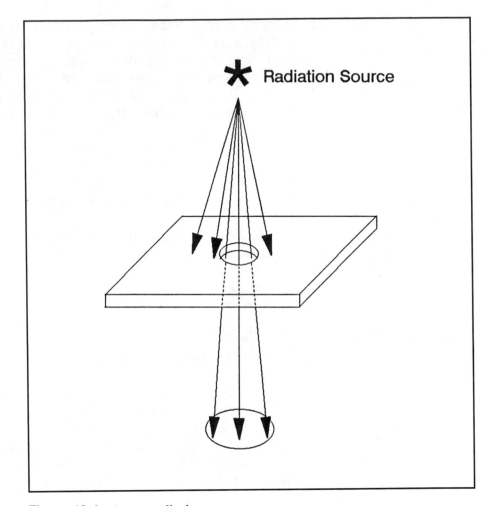

Figure 12-1. Aperture diaphragm

base and tip), Figure 12-2. These devices—available in a variety of lengths and diameters—can be inserted and interchanged under the X-ray tube window to accommodate various film sizes and source-to-image distances.
Collimators. A collimator, often referred to as a variable collimator, is an efficient beam-limitation device. Attached to the radiographic tube housing, the collimator looks like a square box with a clear plastic window. It contains two sets of adjustable lead shutters mounted at different levels, a light source, and a mirror to deflect the light source. The lead

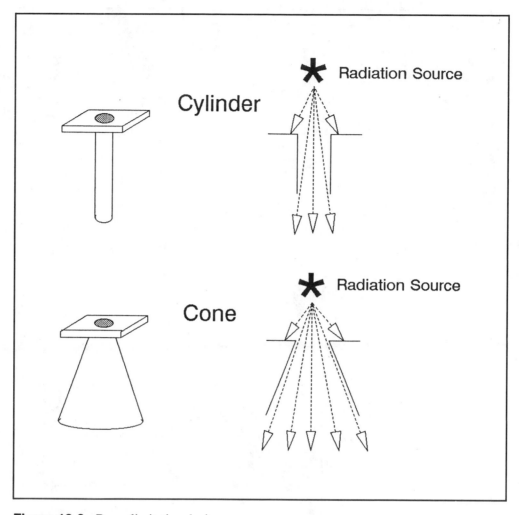

Figure 12-2. Beam-limitation devices

shutters can be adjusted so as to limit the primary radiation beam to the area of clinical interest, Figure 12-3.

Proper collimation of the primary radiation beam will result in an unexposed margin around the edge of the radiograph. Never allow the primary radiation beam to expose an area beyond the area of clinical interest. The examples in Figure 12-4 illustrate proper and improper collimation technique.

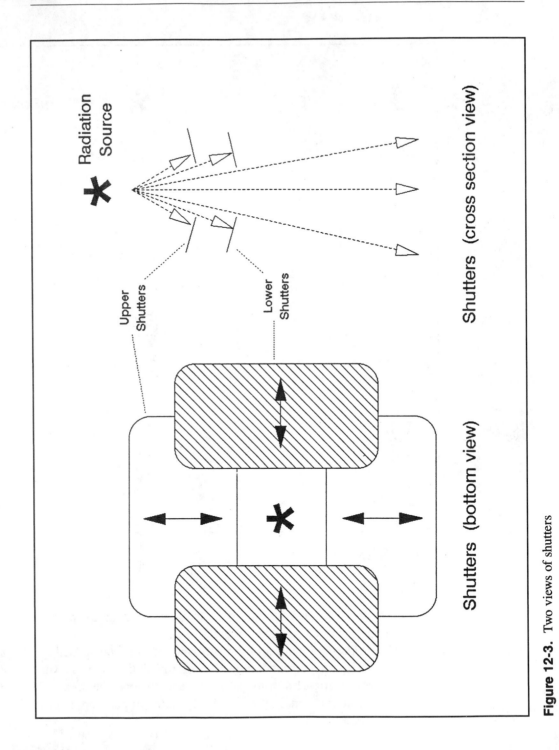

Figure 12-3. Two views of shutters

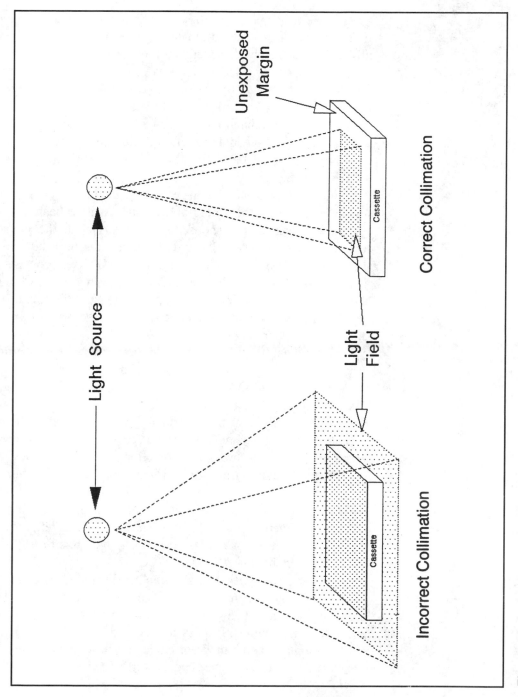

Figure 12-4. Proper use of collimation

The collimator is equipped with a light source that simulates the radiation exposure area. The collimator light is used as a guide in positioning, alignment, central ray placement, and collimation. If the light source becomes out of alignment with the actual area of radiation exposure, errors in positioning, alignment, central ray placement, or collimation may occur. Daily use, a bump, or jarring of the collimator housing may result in misalignment. The radiographer should include a collimator-light-source-accuracy check as part of a scheduled routine equipment-maintenance check. Whenever in doubt about the collimator-light-source accuracy, perform a light-source-accuracy check.

The efficiency of any beam-restricting device depends upon its regular and proper use by the radiographer. The positive beam limitation (PBL) system was designed in response to the concern about the operator forgetting to limit the beam. The PBL system actually restricts the primary beam to the film size used in the bucky tray. The PBL system consists of electronic sensors installed in the bucky tray holder. When a film holder is locked into the bucky tray, the electronic sensors transmit the film size information to the collimator which automatically adjusts the primary beam to the size of the film holder, Figure 12-5.

An additional benefit of restricting the primary beam is improved radiographic quality. A properly collimated primary radiation beam produces less secondary scattered radiation, thus reducing possible film fog or increased film darkening.

Filtration. Filtration of the primary radiation beam is another method used to protect the patient from unnecessary radiation exposure. Radiographic filters serve two major functions by removing low-energy, long-wavelength photons from the primary beam. These functions are to 1) protect the patients' skin and superficial tissue and 2) improve the quality of the radiation beam. By removing the longer wavelengths, the beam is more homogeneous in wavelength. This filtering is referred to as attenuation of the beam. Ultimately, as primary radiation is restricted and filtered, there is less radiation to scatter.

There are two types of radiographic filtration: inherent filtration and added filtration. Inherent filtration consists of the tube's glass envelope, insulating oil, and the glass window. Inherent filtration is expressed in equivalent aluminum thickness and should be at least 0.5 mm of aluminum. Aluminum is the metal of choice because it effectively removes long wavelengths, is inexpensive, and is sturdy.

Figure 12-5. Positive beam limitation (PBL) device. The radiation beam is properly limited from the source (tube) to the cassette.

Added filtration is any filtration added to the existing inherent filtration. These filters, usually consisting of aluminum sheets, may be added outside the tube housing. The inherent filtration plus added filtration represent the required amount of total filtration. The amount of total radiographic-tube filtration is dependent upon the kilovoltage ranges of the equipment, e.g., 50–70 kVp = 1.5 mm aluminum; above 70 kVp = 2.5 mm aluminum.

Gonadal Shielding. Gonadal shielding protects the patients' gonads from direct primary exposure by placing shielding material between the X-ray beam and the patients' gonads. Gonadal shielding should be used in addition to primary beam restriction and never as a substitute for it.

Gonad shielding should be provided for all persons having reproductive potential and includes adults of reproductive age and children. The anatomic location of the testes allows for adequate shielding while not obscuring needed clinical information. The ovaries, however, located near the vertebral spine, ureters, and small and large intestines do not permit adequate shielding without obscuring a great deal of anatomy nearby.

The two kinds of gonadal shields are *shadow shields* and *contact shields*. Shadow shields are so named because of the shadow cast by the shields. These shields are suspended from the beam-limiting system. They can be positioned to hang over the patients' gonads and are positioned with the assistance of a light localizer. Contact shields may be flat, uncontoured, lead-impregnated material placed on or taped to the patient to cover the gonads, or they may be shaped and contoured to enclose the male reproductive organs, Figure 12-6.

Flat contact shields are most effective for anterior-posterior or posterior-anterior projections when the patient is recumbent. Flat contact shields can be easily used for male and female patients; whereas the shaped contact shield is designed exclusively for use with male patients.

Shaped contact shields are used with disposable supporters. The cup-shaped shield permits enclosure of the scrotum and penis and remains in place with the patient in an upright or recumbent position.

Gonadal shields should meet the following specifications based on the kVp range used:

0.25 mm lead equivalent for 100 kVp or less
0.5 mm lead equivalent for 100–150 kVp
1.0 mm lead equivalent for 150 kVp and above

The decision to use gonadal shielding must be considered with each individual patient's situation and the radiographic request. However, the following criteria provide guides for deciding when gonadal shielding should be used:

1. Use gonadal shielding on all patients who have a reasonable likelihood of reproducing.
2. Use gonadal shielding on all children.

Figure 12-6. Examples of gonadal shields *(Courtesy of General Electric Medical Systems)*

3. Use gonadal shielding if the gonads lie within the primary beam or within 5 cm (2½ in) of the primary beam's edge.
4. Use gonadal shielding if the shielding will not obscure (cover) necessary diagnostic information on the radiograph.

Gonadal shields can develop cracks and pinpoint holes with constant use or if improperly stored. Gonadal shields should be stored flat without folds when not in use and should be regularly checked for cracks or pinpoint holes that can allow radiation leaks to the patient.

Technical Factor Selection. Selection of the correct combination of technical factors has a direct impact on the amount of radiation received by the patient. Table 12-4 lists technical factors and their roles in radiation protection.

PREGNANT PATIENT

Observing all radiation-protection guidelines is extremely important if the patient is pregnant or a pregnancy is suspected. It is important to remember that it is the doctor's responsibility to evaluate the patient and to determine if the diagnostic benefits outweigh the risks associated with radiation exposure. The radiographer's responsibility is to avoid unnecessary radiation exposure and to produce diagnostic-quality radiographs while providing for patient comfort and safety. This can be accomplished by performing all recommended radiation-protection guidelines and by providing the pregnant patient with a lead apron or shield placed over the uterus or totally surrounding the pelvis, Figure 12-7.

Radiation-protection procedures for the potentially pregnant patient conforms to the ALARA concept. The use of the so-called "ten day rule," which stated that pelvic or abdominal examinations of women of childbearing age be done only in the first ten days following the onset of menstruation, is no longer used. The guideline to follow is that *all* radiographic

TABLE 12–4 TECHNICAL FACTORS/ROLES	
FACTOR	**EFFECT**
Exposure selection of high kVp and low mAs	Reduces radiation dose
Proper film processing	Reduces repeat examinations
Use of a grid	Improves radiographic quality
Use of intensifying screen	Reduces amount of radiation exposure required Reduces patient radiation dose
Reduction of repeat examinations	Reduces radiation dose

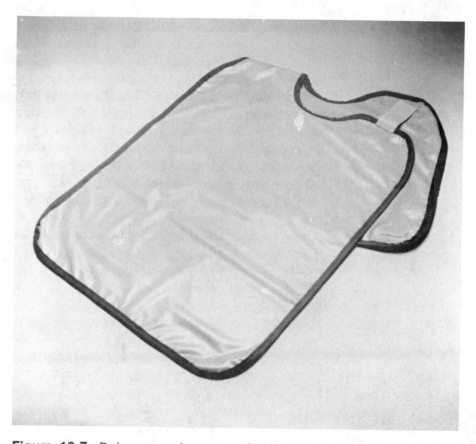

Figure 12-7. Patient protective apron *(Courtesy of General Electric Medical Systems)*

procedures be performed to keep the radiation exposure as low as reasonably achievable.

Although the major responsibility for patient radiation safety rests with the doctor and radiation operator, the current trend in consumer awareness and involvement focuses some responsibility to the patient. This responsibility involves the patient being aware and asking questions about medical care and adopting a personal philosophy of not requesting diagnostic radiographic procedures when alternative diagnostic measures are suggested by the attending physician. The United States Food and Drug Administration has responded to this new focus on consumer awareness by developing an X-ray record card similar to immunization record cards.

RADIATION-PROTECTION PROCEDURES FOR THE OPERATOR

Cardinal Principles

There are three cardinal principles of radiation protection: *t*ime, *d*istance, and *s*hielding (TDS), Figure 12-8. If used together, the principles of TDS can minimize radiation exposure to the patient and radiographer. These three cardinal principles were developed for nuclear-energy employees who have the potential to be exposed to high levels of radiation in their workplace. The radiographer, of course, is not expected to be employed in a high-level radiation area, such as a nuclear energy plant, but the cardinal principles have practical application to medical radiography.

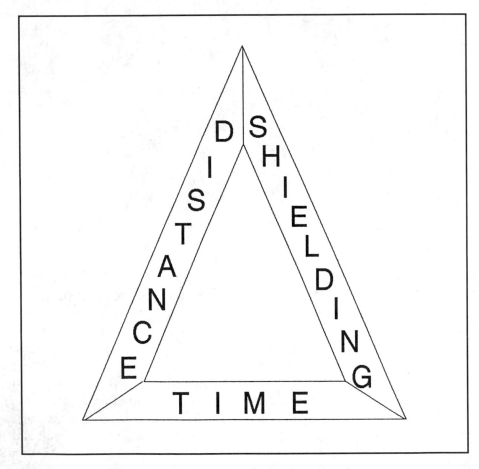

Figure 12-8. Three cardinal principles of radiation protection

Time.   Radiation exposure is proportional to the amount of time spent in the radiation. A five-minute exposure to radiation would result in a radiation dose five times as great as a one-minute exposure to radiation. This has several implications that can be related to the radiographer and the patient:

1. A radiographer should reduce the amount of time exposed to radiation. Do not stay in a radiography room during the exposure unless you are standing behind a protective barrier.
2. A radiographer should reduce the amount of time that the patient is exposed to radiation. Reduce retake examinations and subsequently reduce time and radiation exposure.
3. The radiographer should use a fast exposure-time factor whenever possible. A fast exposure time can reduce radiographic motion unsharpness due to patient movement.

Distance.   Distance between the radiographer and the radiation source is a very effective way to reduce radiation exposure and the most easily applied principle of radiation protection. The inverse square law which applies to point sources of radiation can be used to demonstrate the effect of distance on radiation intensity, Figure 12-9. Radiation from an X-ray tube is considered to be a point source. Radiation intensity, from a point source, varies inversely as the square of the distance from the source.

X-rays are like light in that the further you move away from the source, the dimmer the light becomes or the less intense the X rays become. Figure 12-9 demonstrates that doubling the distance in an X-ray exposure will spread the radiation over four (4) times the original area size; however, the radiation will have only one-fourth its original intensity. Distance is a very important safety guideline because operator protection increases as the distance from the radiation source is increased. For example, as the distance doubles from the radiation source, the operator gains four times more protection because the radiation intensity is decreased by one-fourth its original intensity.

The distance principle as applied to patient protection means that every radiographic examination should be performed with the X-ray tube positioned at the proper SID from the patient or part being examined.

Shielding.   Shielding is the third cardinal principle of radiation protection. As X-ray photons travel through the air or through an absorber (such as living tissue), the quantity and energy of the X-ray photons decrease.

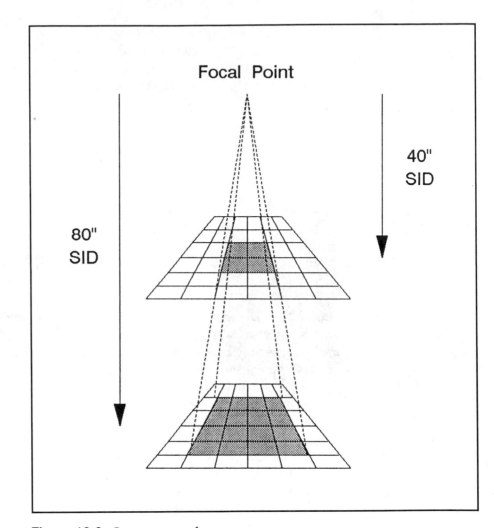

Figure 12-9. Inverse square law

The degree to which the quantity and energy of the X-ray photons are decreased depends upon several factors: 1) original quantity and energy of the X-ray beam; 2) type of absorber material; and 3) thickness of the absorber material. If X-ray photons travel through enough absorbing material, eventually their energy will be lost to the material and no X rays will emerge through to the other side.

Protective shields are usually constructed of lead or a concrete wall barrier. This serves as an absorber of the radiation and should be situated so that it intercepts the primary radiation and any radiation that has scattered.

The radiographer should stand behind a lead shield or wall barrier when making the radiographic exposure. The radiographer should not peek around the shield or wall to watch the patient but should watch the patient through the protective glass window installed in the shield or wall, Figure 12-10.

Figure 12-10. Arrangement of a control console of an X-ray machine with protective leaded wall and window (*Courtesy of General Electric Medical Systems*)

Protective Apparel

Protective apparel is used for patient or operator protection whenever additional protection is desired or necessary. Protective apparel consists of lead-impregnated vinyl gloves and apron, Figure 12-11. The lead gloves and apron should be at least 0.25 mm lead equivalency when radiographing at normal operating voltages. Handle lead aprons, gloves, and gonad shields with care. Protective apparel should be properly stored when not in use to prevent cracks from developing in the lead. Do not store the items by folding since cracks could result from the bending of the protective lead insert. Cracks could permit radiation to leak through.

The lead apron and gloves should be checked for cracks once every three months.

Figure 12-11. Use of lead apron and gloves for personal protection *(Courtesy of General Electric Medical Systems)*

The Pregnant Radiographer

A radiation operator who becomes pregnant while employed in that capacity should discuss her pregnancy with her supervisor and attending physician. These three persons should review together all radiation-protection guidelines. The dose equivalent is 5 mSv (0.5 rem) for the total period of the pregnancy and 0.5 mSv (0.05 rem) for any given month. Remember, the first trimester (first three months) is the most critical period of fetal development, and it is recommended that the pregnant radiographer receive as little radiation exposure as possible.

Optional protective measures that a pregnant radiographer may use include wearing a protective lead apron of at least 0.5 mm lead in addition to standing behind the protective barrier and wearing a "Baby" film badge. The "Baby" film badge may be worn in addition to the operator film badge. The badge worn near the hip or pelvic area should be labeled as "Baby" badge so that a separate record can be maintained.

If a pregnant radiographer performs the usual recommended radiation safety procedures during all radiography examinations and uses the optional protective measures outlined, it is nearly impossible to come close to the fetal dose equivalent. Pregnancy does not justify a lay-off or termination of employment.

RADIATION DETECTION AND MONITORING

Accurate radiation detection and measurement is necessary if occupational exposure levels are to be kept below the maximum-permissible-dose levels. Personnel and area monitoring are the most commonly used procedures used to determine occupational exposure.

Personnel Monitoring Devices

Personnel monitoring provides important information regarding the amount of radiation exposure received by an operator. The information gathered from personnel monitoring must then be reviewed to determine if it is within the maximum-permissible-dose guidelines. After the review, corrective actions may be required to reduce or eliminate the radiation exposure. It should be recognized that personnel radiation monitoring is just that—a monitor that records the amount of radiation received and is an indication of the radiographer's working habits and working conditions. One should never assume one is safe just because monitoring is occurring. Nor should it be assumed that because no exposure has ever been recorded, no exposure has ever been or ever will be received. Also, personnel monitoring devices record only the exposure received in the area in which they are worn. The device should be attached to the front of the clothing so it records the radiation received by the radiation operator's body trunk. During fluoroscopic procedures when the operator wears a protective lead apron, an additional monitoring device may be worn outside of the protective apron at the collar level to record exposure to the radiosensitive organs of the head, neck, and lens of the eye.

There are three basic kinds of personnel-radiation-monitoring devices: film badges, thermoluminescent dosimeters, and pocket ionization chambers. Usually, the nature of the occupation and the type of ionizing radiation will determine the choice of personnel monitoring device. A summary of personnel monitoring devices is presented in Table 12-5.

Film Badges.   Film badges are the most frequently used type of personnel monitoring device. They are economical and considered relatively accurate in recording low doses of radiation if instructions regarding care and use are followed.

A film badge consists of three parts: a film packet, metal filters, and a plastic holder with a clip attachment, Figure 12-12. The plastic holder is made of a low-atomic-number material so that low-energy radiation may reach the film packet. Metal filters of aluminum or copper are contained in the plastic holder and allow for measurement of the radiation energy reaching the film packet. After processing, the degree of film darkening beneath the filters provides a basis for estimating the radiation exposure. A densitometer is used to measure film density and then compared to the exposure value of a control film of similar density on a characteristic curve. In addition to the amount of radiation received, the information provided by film-badge films also includes: 1) direction of the radiation exposure (from front to back or from back to front) and 2) whether exposure was from excessive scattered radiation or a single primary beam exposure.

The radiographic-film packet consists of radiation dosimetry film and is similar in size and shape to dental film. Enclosed in a light-free envelope, the radiographic film has sensitivity to doses ranging from 0.1 mSv (10 millirems) to 5 Sv (500 rems). The light-free envelope has a lead foil back that absorbs scatter radiation from behind the device.

Film-badge film packets must be returned to the monitoring company at specific intervals (usually once a month) for processing. The monitoring company provides a control film packet with each shipment of film pack-

TABLE 12-5 SUMMARY OF PERSONNEL MONITORING DEVICES

DEVICE	ADVANTAGES	DISADVANTAGES
Film Badge	• Economical, low-cost • Durable container • Permanent record of personnel exposure • Detects both small and large exposures • Filters allow determination regarding direction of exposure and cause of exposure (scatter/primary) • Control badge provided • Reliable with X-ray and gamma radiation and differentiates between	• Only effective if worn and cared for according to monitoring company directions • Records exposure only in area where badge is worn • Film packet can be fogged by excessive temperature or humidity
TLD Device	• Accurately records dose • Not sensitive to excessive temperature or humidity • May be worn up to three months	• Initial high cost • No permanent record of readings • Not effective if not worn • Person performing readout must follow recommended procedures
Pocket Ionization Chamber	• Easy to wear • Sensitive and accurately records dose • Immediate readout in self-reading chambers	• Expensive • No permanent record of readings • Chamber should be read and recharged daily • Not effective if not worn

Figure 12-12. Typical film badge and holder

ets. The control film packet serves as a control for comparing the worn film packets after they have been returned for processing. The control film packet must be stored in a radiation-free area within the medical facility.

Monitoring companies provide a written report containing the results for each film packet and the control packet. These film-badge reports should be reviewed by the facility's radiation safety officer or supervisor to determine compliance with MPD guidelines and corrective action taken as necessary. The badge reports should be permanently maintained with personnel records.

Although film badges have the advantage of being economical and not easily damaged if dropped, the disadvantages must be considered. The film packet is sensitive to extreme temperature and humidity levels and is not accurate over long periods of recording time, generally not longer than one month.

Thermoluminescent Dosimeters. A thermoluminescent dosimeter (TLD) badge is similar in appearance to the film badge; however, it contains a different type of monitoring system. Special crystals in the TLD undergo physical property changes when struck by ionizing radiation. When heated, the crystals emit energy in the form of visible light, equal to the amount of radiation exposure absorbed. A TLD analyzer is then used to heat and measure the amount of radiation received. TLD monitoring devices have several advantages that film badges do not have. They give more accurate recording of low radiation doses; they are less sensitive to extreme temperatures or humidity; and they can be used for up to three months. Disadvantages include initial high cost and no permanent record of the radiation reading since the readout process destroys the stored information.

Pocket Ionization Chambers. The most sensitive, yet infrequently used, personnel monitoring device in diagnostic radiology is the pocket ionization chamber. The pocket dosimeter resembles a fountain pen and contains an ionization chamber, which may be either a self-reading type or a non-self-reading chamber (which requires the use of a special electrometer accessory for a readout).

One advantage of the pocket ionization chamber is that the self-reading type can provide an immediate exposure readout. This is an important and critical feature often required by those who work in high-radiation-exposure occupations. These chambers are expensive and require careful attention to the manufacturer's directions during the readout.

Survey Instruments for Area Monitoring

Radiation survey instruments are used to detect the presence or absence of radiation in a particular area. Generally, medical radiographers will not be required to use survey instruments to determine radiation exposure; however, it is important to recognize the function of these instruments. The Geiger-Müller (G-M) detector, ionization chamber-type survey meter, and the proportional counter are gas-filled radiation survey instruments used to detect radiation and its exposure quantity. The Victoreen condenser R-meter used to calibrate radiography equipment is also a gas-filled ionization chamber. Survey instruments are commonly used by radiation physicists, equipment inspectors, radiography service people, and others who are employed in nuclear occupations where environmental radiation exposure may occur.

REVIEW QUESTIONS

1. The main goal of all radiation protection procedures
   a) is to reduce radiation exposure to zero
   b) allows exposures up to the maximal limits
   c) is to limit only nonoccupational exposures
   d) is to keep all radiation exposures as low as reasonably achievable
2. The annual effective dose equivalent for whole-body occupational exposure is
   a) 5 mSv (0.5 rem)
   b) 50 mSv (5 rem)
   c) 150 mSv (15 rem)
   d) 500 mSv (50 rem)
3. The annual effective dose equivalent for embryo-fetus exposure to term is
   a) 5 mSv (0.5 rem)
   b) 50 mSv (5 rem)
   c) 150 mSv (15 rem)
   d) 500 mSv (50 rem)
4. The annual effective dose equivalent for infrequent, nonoccupational exposure is
   a) 5 mSv (0.5 rem)
   b) 50 mSv (5 rem)
   c) 150 mSv (15 rem)
   d) 500 mSv (50 rem)
5. The cumulative lifetime exposure for a fifty-year-old radiation worker is
   a) 5 mSv (0.5 rem)
   b) 50 mSv (5 rem)
   c) 150 mSv (15 rem)
   d) 500 mSv (50 rem)
6. Which of the following areas can contribute to reducing patient radiation exposure?
   1) patient communication

2) patient preparation
3) primary beam limitation
   a) 1 and 2
   b) 1 and 3
   c) 2 and 3
   d) 1, 2, and 3

7. Methods of limiting the primary beam include
  1) aperture diaphragm
  2) cone
  3) collimator
   a) 1 and 2
   b) 1 and 3
   c) 2 and 3
   d) 1, 2, and 3

8. Which of the following is true?
  1) Increasing distance increases radiation exposure.
  2) Decreasing exposure time decreases radiation exposure.
  3) Increasing shielding decreases radiation exposure.
   a) 1 and 2
   b) 1 and 3
   c) 2 and 3
   d) 1, 2, and 3

9. Some advantages of using a film badge for personnel monitoring include
  1) low cost
  2) reliability
  3) not sensitive to excessive humidity or temperature
   a) 1 and 2
   b) 1 and 3
   c) 2 and 3
   d) 1, 2, and 3

10. Some advantages of using a thermoluminescent dosimeter (TLD) for personnel monitoring include
  1) low cost
  2) accuracy
  3) not sensitive to excessive humidity or temperature
   a) 1 and 2
   b) 1 and 3
   c) 2 and 3
   d) 1, 2, and 3

Glossary

Absorbed dose the amount of radiation energy absorbed in tissue; measured in greys

Acute dose the amount of radiation received in a single exposure

ALARA concept as low as reasonably achievable; the idea that radiation exposures be kept as low as possible

Alpha particle a product of radioactive decay composed of two protons and two neutrons; a helium nucleus

Ampere the S.I. base unit of electrical current; also expressed as 1 coulomb/second

Amplitude the fluctuation of a wave above or below the normal non-perturbed state

Anion a negatively charged particle

Anode the positively charged side of an electrical circuit; the target side of an x-ray tube

Aperture diaphragm an x-ray beam restrictor consisting of a lead sheet with a hole

Apnea cessation of breathing

Apparent focal spot the size of the projected x-ray tube focal spot

Area the amount of enclosed space; height times width; measured in cm^2

Asymptomatic without symptoms of disease or illness

Atom the smallest particle that an element can be reduced to while still maintaining its chemical identity

Atomic mass number the number of protons and neutrons in a nucleus

Atomic number the number of protons in a nucleus

Automatic exposure x-ray exposure timing determined by a phototimer or similar device

Autonomy freedom to govern one's self or self-governance

Autotransformer a transformer consisting of two windings on a single core; used in x-ray machines to change the line voltage

Axilla the region under the shoulder, commonly referred to as the armpit

Background radiation the normal amount of radiation exposure expected from unavoidable natural and artificial sources

Beam restriction control of the field size of an x-ray beam

Becquerel the S.I. of radioactivity; equal to one disintegration per second

Beneficience   in health care, a duty to others to provide or improve conditions that promote physical and emotional well-being

Beta particle   a product of radioactive decay physically identical to an electron

Biomedical ethics   ethics applied to the knowledge of modern medical technologies

Body language   nonverbal indicators of communication, e.g., smiling, frowning, clenched fists

Calcium tungstate   a material developed by Thomas A. Edison and used in intensifying screens

Cassette   a rigid holder that contains intensifying screens; used to hold film

Cathode   the negatively charged side of an electrical circuit; the side of an x-ray tube where electrons are produced

Cation   a positively charged particle

Cheyne-Stokes   abnormal breathing in which apnea (cessation of breathing) occurs from 10–60 seconds

Circuit breaker   a device used to quickly shut down an electrical circuit in case of overload

Classical scatter   an interaction of an x-ray photon with an atom that results in a change of direction of the photon with no loss of energy

Collimator   an adjustable x-ray beam restrictor

Compound   a substance composed of like molecules

Compton effect   an interaction of an x-ray photon with an atom that results in scattered, lower energy photon and an electron

Conductor   a material that carries electricity easily

Cone   a conical shaped x-ray beam restrictor

Confidentiality   a patient's legal and ethical right to privacy

Consumer-Patient Radiation Safety Act   enacted in 1981, it gives Congress the power to protect consumers and patients from unnecessary or excessive radiation exposure

Contact shield   a protective radiation shield that is in physical contact with the patient

Continuing education unit (CEU)   a unit of education usually designed to provide a review or update of technical information to credentialed individuals

Contrast   differences seen between body organs and tissue thicknesses; controlled by kVp

Coulomb the S.I. unit of electrical charge; one A · s

Curie the obsolete unit of radioactivity; equal to 3.7×10^{10} disintegrations per second

Current the flow of electrons in an electrical circuit

Density overall blackness of the radiographic image; controlled by mAs

Diastolic the phase of the cardiac cycle in which the heart muscle is at rest

Diode an electrical device that allows the flow of electricity in one direction only

Distortion variation from normal shape; a misshapen radiographic image

DNA deoxyribo nucleic acid; the biomolecule that carries genetic information

Dose rate the amount of radiation delivered per unit time; can be measured in sieverts per minute

Dyspnea difficult or labored breathing

Effective dose equivalent the total radiation exposure of a human

Effective focal spot the size of the focal spot that is perceived on the film

Electric potential the ability of electricity to do work; measured in volts

Electricity the presence or movement of charged particles

Electrification imparting a charge to objects

Electrodynamics the movement of electrical charge

Electromagnetic radiation radiation consisting of an electrical component and a magnetic component; described in terms of energy, wavelength, and frequency

Electron a negatively charged fundamental particle found in atomic orbitals

Electron binding energy the amount of energy holding an electron in its orbital

Electrostatics attraction or repulsion due to electrical charge

Element a chemically distinguishable substance consisting of only one kind of atom

Empathy the ability to understand another's situation, such as fear, pain, anger, without actually having the emotion

Energy the ability to do work; usually divided into kinetic energy, the energy of motion, and potential energy, the energy of position; measured in joules

Ethics the philosophical study of human behavior or conduct

Febrile   having elevated body temperature; feverish

Filament   the heated wire in the cathode of an x-ray tube where electrons are produced

Filament current   the amount of electrical current flowing through the filament of an x-ray tube; measured in amperes

Film badge   a personnel radiation monitor that measures radiation exposure by use of film

Film fog   "undesirable" density (film darkening); obscures image details

Filter   a metal device used to attenuate x rays

Filtration   the use of a filter to attenuate x rays

Fluorescence   a type of luminescence or "lighting up" that occurs when certain phosphors (calcium tungstate) absorb radiation

Focal spot (FS)   the region of the x-ray tube target where the electron beam is focused

Focusing cup   the metal cup surrounding the filament in an x-ray tube that focuses an x-ray beam

Fomite   an object that has been contaminated with a pathogen and serves to spread disease

Fractionation   an x-ray exposure in multiple doses repeated over a period of time

Frequency   the repetition rate of electromagnetic radiation; measured in hertz

Full-wave rectification   a type of rectification that utilizes both halves of the AC voltage pulse

Gamma rays   high-energy electromagnetic radiation resulting from radioactive decay of a nucleus

Genetic effect   the ability of ionizing radiations to damage reproductive cells

Geometric factors   factors of distance and positioning that affect the radiographic quality

Gonadal shield   a radiation shield used to protect the reproductive organs

Gray   the S.I. unit of radiation absorbed dose; also expressed as joules per kilogram

Grid   a radiographic accessory constructed with lead strips to reduce the amount of scattered radiation from a given exposure reaching the film

Half-value layer (HVL)   the amount of material needed to attenuate a radiation beam by 50%

Half-wave rectification a type of rectification that utilizes only one half of the AC voltage pulse

Heat unit (HU) a measure of the heat accumulated in the anode of an x-ray tube due to self-absorption in the anode

Heel effect diminished x-ray intensity at the anode end of an x-ray tube due to self-absorption in the anode

Hertz the S.I. unit of frequency; expressed as 1/s

High voltage transformer the transformer in an x-ray machine circuit that steps up the voltage prior to use in the x-ray tube

Hypertension an elevation in blood pressure that is influenced by conditions, diseases, emotional, and environmental stress

Hyperventilation increased respiratory rate or breathing that is deeper than normal

Hypotension a decrease in blood pressure

Illuminator (viewbox) a metal framework housing fluorescent tubes that emit light of standard daylight color and intensity

Image shape the true shape of the anatomy projected onto the film so that there is no distortion or magnification

Impulse timer an x-ray exposure timer that is energized to various time intervals

Inertia the tendency of a moving body to remain in motion or a stationary body to remain at rest

Informed consent an individual's right to disclosure of all information related to a medical procedure or treatment to assure the person's full understanding for voluntary consent to accept medical care

Intensifying screens screens composed of fluorescent phosphors (i.e., calcium tungstate mixed with a binding agent)

International System of Units (SI Units) the approved system of measurement based on the meter, second, kilogram, ampere; also called S.I. units

Ion an electrically charged particle

Ion pair the free electron and charged atom resulting from the ionization of an atom

Ionization the imparting of charge to an atom by the removal or addition of an electron

Ionization chamber a device used to measure the quantity of ionization caused by radiation

Ionizing radiation electromagnetic or particulate radiation that imparts charge to atoms

Isotopes a nuclear arrangement with differing neutron numbers and the same atomic numbers

Justice the balancing and fair distribution of medical care, facilities, and resources for society

Kilogram the S.I. base unit of mass
Kilovolt thousands of volts; the unit used to measure the energy of an x-ray beam
Kilovolt peak (kVp) the maximum voltage in an electrical voltage pulse
Kilovolt peak meter the device that measures the energy of an x-ray beam

Law of Bergonié and Tribondeau the relation of radiation sensitivity to mitotic state and differentiation
Law of conservation of energy the physical principle that energy can neither be created nor destroyed
Length the spatial dimension of an object; measured in meters
Limited radiographer a multi-skilled person dedicated to assisting in many aspects of medical care including basic radiography tasks under the supervision of a licensed practitioner of the healing arts
Line focus principle the effect whereby the apparent focal spot is smaller than the actual focal spot of an x-ray tube
Linear energy transfer (LET) the loss of energy to matter by radiation; measured in keV/?m

Magnetism the ability of certain materials to attract iron and other metals
Magnification enlargement of the size of the actual anatomical part
Mass the quantity of material in an object; measured in kilograms
mAs timer an x-ray machine timer that terminates the exposure when a specific mAs is attained
Matter the substance of an object; composed of atoms
Maximum permissible dose (MPD) the maximum amount of radiation allowed under radiation safety standards; defined for the whole body, body parts, and calendar periods
Meter the S.I. base unit of length
Microorganisms extremely small organisms: bacteria, fungi, protozoa, rickettsiae, and viruses
Milliammeter the instrument used to measure x-ray tube current
Milliamperage (mA) the unit of x-ray tube current

Milliamperage-seconds (mAs) the product of x-ray tube current and exposure time; a measure of x-ray quantity

Molecule chemical combinations of atoms into substances

Momentum the product of mass and velocity

Motion the property of movement

Negligible individual risk level (NIRL) a level of risk that can be dismissed; the risk associated with an annual effective dose equivalent of 0.01 mSv

Neutron an uncharged fundamental particle found in the nucleus of an atom

Nonmaleficience in the health professions, to prevent harm or to cause no harm to another person

Nonpathogenic microorganisms microscopic organisms that are not harmful

Nosocomial infection opportunist infections; a group of pathogenic microorganisms that are common in medical settings

Nuclear energy energy produced by fission or fusion of an atomic nucleus

Nucleus 1) the center of an atom containing neutrons and protons; 2) the portion of a cell containing the DNA

Object image distance (OID) distance between the part being examined and the film

Ohm the S.I. unit of electrical resistance

Ohm's law the physical principle which states that voltage is the product of current and resistance

Orbital the preferred energy level in an atom for an electron

Overexposure too much exposure of the film; usually too much density

Particulate radiation ionizing radiation consisting of physical particles such as electrons or neutrons

Passbox a light-tight passageway between the darkroom and outside areas. Allows passage to darkroom while preventing light from entering

Pathogenic organisms microscopic organisms that are harmful and capable of causing disease

Penumbra geometric blur (fuzziness) of the anatomical part being examined in the radiographic image

Philosophy learning related to a search for truth and a general understanding of values and reality

Photoelectric effect   an interaction of an x-ray photon with an atom that results in the absorption of the x-ray and the emission of an electron

Photographic effect (PE)   effect of radiation or light on the emulsion of the film; quality of the image

Photographic factors   factors that control the black and white radiographic image; density (mAs) and contrast (kVp)

Photons   the massless particles that convey electromagnetic force; x rays and light

Phototimer   an x-ray machine time that terminates the exposure after absorption of a preset amount of radiation

Positive beam limitation (PBL)   a device that collimates an x-ray beam according to the size of the film cassette

Potential difference   the difference in voltage in an electrical circuit

Power   the amount of work done per unit time; measured in watts

Primary circuit   the part of an x-ray machine circuit on the input side of the high voltage transformer

Professional   a highly skilled person; a person trained in the liberal arts or sciences and also possessing advanced education and training

Professional ethics   in the health related professions, standards of conduct that relate to duties and obligations of health care practitioners

Proton   a positively charged fundamental particle found in the nucleus of an atom

Protraction   a radiation exposure that occurs over a prolonged period of time

Rad   the obsolete unit of radiation absorbed dose

Radiation   electromagnetic waves or particular matter emitted as a result of electronic or atomic transitions

Radioactive decay (disintegration)   the release of radiation by an unstable nucleus

Radiographic artifact   areas of increased or decreased fim darkening (density) on radiographs

Radiologic technologist   a person who has completed an approved educational program and passed an examination administered by the American Registry of Radiology Technologists

Radiosensitivity   the measure of the response of a biological organism to radiation

Rare-earth screens   screens composed of elements that belong to Group III in the periodic table of elements and have atomic numbers between 57 and 71

Reciprocity   law that states that response of film to radiation of a given intensity will remain unchanged if the milliamperage and time factors are equal

Rectifier   an electrical device that allows the flow of electricity in one direction only

Relative biologic effectiveness (RBE)   a measure of the biological effects of different types of radiations; the ratio of the effect of a standard radiation to a test radiation

Rem   roentgen equivalent mammal; the obsolete unit of dose equivalent

Remnant radiation   after partial absorption of the primary beam, remnant radiation is the energy that penetrates and emerges from the anatomy or object being examined and reaches the film emulsion

Resistance   the property of a material that impedes the flow of electricity; measured in ohms

Resistance resolution   ability of a system of screens and film to produce and record the image of a part of human anatomy

Roentgen, Wilhelm Conrad   discovered x rays in 1895

Safelight illumination   incandescent lamps with a colored filter which allows light to be transmitted in the darkroom without fogging the film

Scattered radiation   the secondary radiation produced as a result of interactions of the primary radiation beam with atoms

Screen lag (afterglow)   phosphorescence or the presence of light or "glow" emitted by phosphors in an intensifying screen after the x-ray exposure has ceased

Second   the S.I. base unit of time

Secondary circuit   the part of an x-ray machine circuit on the output side of the high voltage transformer

Secondary radiation   electrons and scattered x rays produced by x-ray interactions with atoms

Sensitometry   study of how radiographic film responds to radiation exposure photographically and to processing conditions chemically

Shadow shield   a radiation shield held or suspended above the patient

Sievert   the S.I. unit of dose equivalent; also expressed as one joule per kilogram

Silver halide crystals active ingredient of the radiographic film emulsion

Silver recovery a chemical or electrolytic process used to remove silver from radiographic fixer solution

Somatic effect effect of radiation on the human body other than the gonads; responsible for cancer and cataracts

Source-to-image distance (SID) distance from the tube (focal spot) to the film

Step-down transformer a transformer that reduces voltage

Step-up transformer a transformer that increases voltage

Sympathy acknowledgment of another person's grief, hurt, or loss

Symptomatic having symptoms of disease or illness

Synchronous timer an x-ray machine timer controlled and driven by an electrical motor

Systolic the phase of the cardiac cycle in which the heart muscle contracts

Target 1) the portion of an anode struck by the electron beam; 2) a radiation-sensitive cellular component

Target theory the theory which states that there are one or two critical targets for radiation damage in a cell

Temperature the amount of thermal kinetic energy in an object; measured in degrees celsius

Thermionic emission the production of electrons by the heating of the x-ray tube filament

Thermoluminescent dosimeter a personnel radiation monitoring device, which, when heated, produces light proportional to the radiation exposure

Time the period when something occurs; measured in seconds

Transformer an electrical device that increases the electrical voltage of a circuit

Tube current the quantity of electrons flowing from the cathode to the anode; measured in mA

Tube rating charts charts that detail safe combination of x-ray tube operating kVp, mA, and exposure time

Umbra sharply (geometrically) defined edges of the anatomical part examined in the radiographic image

Underexposure radiographic image that is too light; usually not enough density

Vector   an infected insect or animal that passes disease through a bite, e.g., ticks, fleas, lice

Velocity   the rate of motion of an object; measured in meters per second

Volt   the S.I. unit of electrical potential difference

Voltage compensator   a device in an x-ray machine circuit that corrects for fluctuations in line voltage

Volume   the amount of space contained in an object; measured in m³

Watt   the S.I. unit of power; also expressed as joules per second

Wave   a periodic disturbance in a substance

Wavelength   the distance between two similar portions of a wave

Work   the expenditure of energy

X ray   a high energy, high frequency, short wavelength electromagnetic radiation

Appendix

TASKS

TASK 2-1

Using "I" Messages

Objective: To recognize and practice using common "I" messages.
Directions: Review the "I" message information, then write your "I" message in the practice activity.

Review Information   Using "I" messages is effective when giving criticism, explaining a problem, making a suggestion, or expressing an opinion. "I" messages don't make others feel offended or put them in a defensive position. There are *two* parts to the "I" message. The *first part* describes your feelings without blaming anyone else for the way you feel.

"YOU" Message (blames others)	"I" Message (first part)
1. "You really make me mad."	1. "I'm feeling upset about this."
2. "You sure are disorganized."	2. "I like to have things well-organized."
3. "You're always interrupting."	3. "Maybe I'm talking too much."
4. "You don't understand."	4. _____
5. "You're walking too fast."	5. _____
6. "You're confusing me."	6. _____
7. "Your smoking bothers me."	7. _____

The *second part* of the "I" message describes how you would like to feel or how you would like the situation to be changed.

"I" Message (describes your feelings)	"I" Message (describes how you would like things to change)
1. "I'm having some difficulty following you."	1. "Could we go back to the first part of your story?"
2. "Although I don't agree, I hear your point of view."	2. "I'd like us to understand each other better."
3. "I'm concerned about the image of our office."	3. "I'm asking everyone to give special attention to personal appearance."

Practice Activities

1. The office staff is having a meeting to decide on a better supply inventory system. Judith insists that she knows the best way and will not give anyone else a chance to talk.

    "YOU" Message: "You're monopolizing the conversation."

    "I" Message, first part: "I appreciate your good ideas."

    "I" Message, second part: "I'd also like to hear some other opinion."

2. Several staff members are eating lunch in the office conference room. In a joking mood, they start to tease you about being the office supervisor's favorite. If your coworkers have a real problem over this, you would like to discuss it.

    "YOU" Message: "If you worked as hard as I do, you might get noticed too."

    "I" Message, first part: _____

    "I" Message, second part: _____

3. You have just started a new job. The supervisor keeps watching everything you do. You would like to be able to work more on your own.

    "YOU" Message: "You're making me nervous."

    "I" Message, first part: _____

    "I" Message, second part: _____

4. Rita collects the money for the coffee fund at work. Everyone is supposed to contribute, and you are the only one who does not drink coffee.

    "YOU" Message: "Rita, you're being unfair. You're the ones who drink the coffee."

    "I" Message, first part: _____

    "I" Message, second part: _____

5. You have noticed that patients often have to wait at the reception area while the receptionist makes appointments. Mrs. Bruce, your supervisor, walks by and you stop to tell her about it.

    "YOU" Message: "Mrs. Bruce, you really need to do somehting about these long lines."

    "I" Message, first part: _____

    "I" Message, second part: _____

TASK 2-2

Using Paraphrasing*

Objective: To recognize and practice using common paraphrasing techniques.

Directions: Review the paraphrasing examples. Read the example statements, then complete the student self-check activity. Write your paraphrasing response.

[Review Information]   Paraphrasing means repeating what a person has said to you, but using slightly different words. Paraphrasing a statement helps you determine whether you understood the message as it was intended. Review the example statements.

Example Statements

Paraphrasing Examples

Patient to Radiographer:
"You know, I took a hard fall and my knee hurts more than the ankle you are X-raying."

Radiographer to Patient:
"*Are you saying* that your knee hurts as much as your ankle?"

Worker to Coworker:
"I want to go to my grandmother's birthday party next Saturday, but I'm afraid to ask for the day off."

Coworker to Worker:
"You sound anxious about asking the supervisor to have the day off."

Worker to Coworker:
"The new sick leave policy is really unfair."

Coworker to Worker:
_____
_____
_____

Patient to Radiographer:
"I'm really dreading the thought of having this chest X ray."

Radiographer to Patient:
_____
_____
_____

Patient to Account Clerk:
"This charge for a chest X ray seems really too high compared to the time it took the girl to take it."

Account Clerk to Patient:
_____
_____
_____
_____

Patient to Radiographer:
"Now I'm going to tell you my old bones hurt and I can't just jump up on that cold table."

Radiographer to Patient:
_____
_____
_____

---

*Adapted from M. M. Brewner, W. C. McMahon, and M. P. Roche. *Job Survival Skills*. New York: Educational Designs, Inc., 1984, p. 65.

TASK 2-3

Using Listening Techniques*

Objective: To recognize personal listening habits.

Directions: Rate your listening habits on the scale below by circling one of the numbers (1–5) after each item.

	Usually	Often	Sometimes	Not Usually	Hardly Ever
1. After only a short period of listening, I start thinking about what I'm going to say next.	1	2	3	4	5
2. If I don't like the person, I don't really listen to what she/he is saying.	1	2	3	4	5
3. I interrupt others before they are finished talking.	1	2	3	4	5
4. I fake attention.	1	2	3	4	5
5. I talk most about myself.	1	2	3	4	5
6. I ask questions.	5	4	3	2	1
7. I give other people a chance to talk.	5	4	3	2	1
8. I try to see things from the other person's point of view.	5	4	3	2	1
9. I maintain good eye contact when listening.	5	4	3	2	1
10. I get so busy taking notes that I miss some of what is said.	5	4	3	2	1
11. I get distracted easily.	5	4	3	2	1
12. I let my mind wander or I daydream when someone is talking.	5	4	3	2	1

ADD THE CIRCLED NUMBERS TO GET YOUR SCORE: _____

45–60   You are a good listener and probably make few mistakes at work. More than likely, people enjoy talking to you and being with you.

31–44   You need to improve your listening skills. This will also improve your job performance.

12–30   You are a poor listener. You have probably lost some friends or made mistakes at work because of your poor listening habits.

Now that you have a score, write out a self-improvement plan of action, if necessary.

---

*Adapted from M. M. Brewner, W. C. McMahon, and M. P. Roche. *Job Survival Skills*. New York: Educational Designs, Inc., 1984, p. 64.

TASK 2-4

Recognizing Barriers to Communication*

Objective: To recognize common barriers to effective communication.
Directions: Read each situation statement and match it to the communication barrier it describes.

Communication Barrier Described

a. Criticizing instead of explaining
b. Poor eye contact
c. Ordering instead of asking politely
d. Interrupting
e. Thinking ahead instead of listening

f. Fear of speaking up
g. Misunderstanding
h. Pretending to listen
i. Ignoring what is said
j. Rudely disagreeing

Situation Statements

_____   1. During break time, several employees were discussing the recent Right to Life protests at the women's clinic. Susan's opinion differed from that of the group. Susan shouted, "You are a bunch of old-fashioned biddies, not liberated." Then she stormed out of the office.

_____ 2. Roger never waits until a person has finished talking. He breaks into conversations with his ideas and never excuses himself.

_____ 3. Rudy was telling Betty about his experience with an angry patient who was upset over a fee for service. Betty looked at Rudy, nodding her head in agreement, but when Rudy asked, "Well what would have said to the patient?" Betty asked, "Rudy, would you repeat what you just said?"

_____ 4. Doctor Parkins told Janna, the medical radiographer, to review the insurance reimbursement on John L. Thomas' X rays. When Janna goes to the files, she finds that Mr. Thomas has had a chest X ray every month for the past year. She wonders if the doctor wants specific information on a particular month or for the entire period.

_____ 5. Supervisor Ellen Brock is giving Marissa directions for opening the office on Saturday. Although she is listening, Marissa is waving to her car-pool companions that she will be out in five minutes.

_____ 6. Robin and Teresa have not been getting along at work. Robin approaches Teresa and says, "I would like to talk with you about our differences." Teresa turns to Helen, another worker, and says, "Where are you going for lunch today?"

_____ 7. Rodney, a limited radiographer, is a new employee and has been asked to perform electrocardiograms (EKG) when he is not busy taking radiographs. Susan has instructed Rodney twice about how to perform an EKG. During an EKG procedure, Rodney has trouble attaching a limb lead and asks Susan for assistance. Susan says, "How many times am I going to have to show you how to do this?"

_____ 8. Joan was telling Becky about her ideas for improving collections on the accounts receivables. Becky keeps thinking, "Wait until she hears my ideas."

_____ 9. Brenda is a new employee in the Springview Medical Clinic. Brenda feels like the clinic supervisor watches every move she makes. This makes Brenda very nervous, but she doesn't know how to tell the supervisor.

_____ 10. Randell, the laboratory assistant, turned from the microscope counter and said, "Jean, get me clean cover slips. I need them right away."

---

*Adapted from M. M. Brewner, W. C. McMahon, and M. P. Roche. _Job Survival Skills_. New York: Educational Designs, Inc., 1984, p. 62–63.

TASK 4-1

Procedure: Hand Washing

Terminal Performance Objective: Provided with soap, nail brush, cuticle stick, paper towels, and a waste receptacle, the student will wash his/her hands. All items on the instructor's checklist must be rated satisfactory or not applicable.

Equipment/Supplies

- Soap (Liquid soap dispenser is recommended; however, students need to know the procedure to follow if bar soap is provided.)
- Hot and cold faucets (Students should recognize the different types of faucets available. Hand operated faucets are a source of contamination for clean hands, so a paper towel should be used to turn off the water. Sinks with foot pedal or elbow levers allow the the water to be turned on, off, and regulated without contamination.)
- Nail brush
- Cuticle stick
- Paper towels
- Waste receptacle (preferably foot operated top opener)

Performance Guide

1. Remove all jewelry: rings, bracelets, watches; wedding rings may be left on, but must be scrubbed.
   Key Point: Jewelry that may harbor bacteria should not be worn during work time. If a sterile procedure requiring donning of gloves is to follow hand washing, rings must be left off until after the procedure is completed.
2. Stand in a comfortable position in front of the sink.
   Key Point: Avoid contaminating the uniform by touching the sink or getting it wet. Usually there are many microorganisms around the sink area, because they grow and multiply rapidly in moist surroundings.
3. Adjust water flow and temperature.
   Key Points: If faucets are hand operated, use paper towel to turn them on. Keep water running continuously throughout the hand-washing procedure.
4. Wet hands thoroughly.
   Key Points: Hold hands down toward sink. Water will drain from wrists to fingertips and carry bacteria away.
5. Apply soap.
   Use approximately one teaspoon of a liquid soap from dispenser.

6. Wash hands.
   a. Use circular motion.
   b. Include palms, wrists, back of hands, and fingers of each hand, using strong friction, Figure Ap.4-1A.

   c. Wash approximately thirty seconds.
   Key Points: Use nail brush on nails and all areas of hands and fingers. Use a cuticle stick to remove any material that the brush may not reach under the nails, Figure Ap.4-1B.

7. Rinse well.
   Key Points: Allow water to run from wrists to fingertips. Avoid touching the inside of the sink.
8. Repeat steps 4–7.
9. Dry hands gently.
10. Turn off water.
    Key Point: If faucets are hand operated, use paper towel to turn off.
    Note: Apply lotion as desired to keep skin soft. Leave the sink and surrounding area neat and dry. A clean, dry environment promotes health.

TASK 4-2

Procedure: Assisting the Falling Patient

Terminal Performance Objective: Provided with a classmate for a patient, assist the falling patient. All items on the instructor's checklist must be marked satisfactory or not applicable.

Equipment/Supplies
■ Classmate as a simulated patient.

Performance Guide

1. Support the patient, holding under the patient's arms. Never try to break the patient's fall because this may increase the possibility of injury.
2. Rest the patient's buttocks against your bent supporting leg.
3. Ease the patient to the floor using the supporting leg.
4. Attend to patient comfort and request assistance.

TASK 4-3

Procedure: Preparing Safety Reports (Accident/Incident)

Terminal Performance Objective: In a simulated safety/accident situation, provided with an accident example and related information, complete a safety and accident report. All items on the instructor's checklist must be rated satisfactory or not applicable.

Equipment/Supplies

■ Accident report form
■ Simulated accident/safety situation (teacher-prepared scene may be used to role play)

Performance Guide

1. Obtain written log or oral report from persons involved.
2. Complete prescribed accident report forms.
3. Verify written report before it is signed by persons involved.
4. Sign and date forms.
5. Forward original and required number of copies to supervisor.
6. File form copy in departmental file.

TASK 4-4

Procedure: Using a Three-Carrier Lift to Transfer the Patient

Terminal Performance Objective: Provided with a classmate for a patient, three classmate assistants, necessary equipment and supplies, use a three-carrier lift to transfer the patient. All items on the instructor's checklist must be marked satisfactory or not applicable.

Equipment/Supplies

■ Classmate as a simulated patient
■ Three assistants
■ Radiographic table
■ Stretcher

Performance Guide

1. Wash hands.
2. Locate and identify the patient.
3. Introduce self and explain procedure.
4. Slide patient to edge of stretcher.
5. Lock stretcher wheels.
6. Position assistants at side of radiographic table:

- one at patient's head and neck
- one at patient's buttocks
- one at legs and ankles

7. Cross patient's arms over chest.
   Persons lifting place their bodies against the area on which patient is lying and place their arms under the patient part they are going to lift.
8. On the count of three, persons lifting roll patient toward their chests.
9. Lifters lift patient and move patient to designated position.
10. Attend to patient comfort.
11. Observe safety precautions.
12. Use good body alignment and mechanics.
13. Repeat procedure in reverse order for transfer back to the stretcher.

TASK 4-5

Procedure: Transferring a Patient Using a Sheet

Terminal Performance Objective: Provided with classmates for a patient and transfer assistants, use a sheet to transfer a patient from a stretcher to the radiographic table. All items on the instructor's checklist must be marked satisfactory or not applicable.

Equipment/Supplies

- Classmate as a simulated patient
- Radiographic table
- Stretcher
- Sheet
- Three to four classmates to serve as transfer assistants.

Performance Guide

1. Wash hands.
2. Explain the procedure to the patient. Talk with the patient. Explain what you will be doing and how he/she can assist.
3. Ask the patient to roll to one side of the stretcher.
4. Fold the sheet in half and place along the patient's backside.
5. Ask the patient to return to his/her back (supine position). The patient will be rolling over the folded sheet.

6. Ask patient to roll to the opposite side (away from the side toward which he/she first rolled).
7. Unfold sheet and smooth out.
8. Ask patient to return to his/her back (supine position).
9. (Need three to four classmates) Position assistant helpers at the following locations:
   - One at patient's head—this person will hold, support, and guide the patient's head during the transfer.
   - One at patient's side.
   - Two across and at side of table onto which patient is to be transferred.
10. All lifters roll transfer sheet up close toward both sides of the patient.
11. In unison, all lifters transfer the patient to the radiographic table.
12. Attend to patient comfort.
13. Observe safety precautions.
14. Use good body alignment and mechanics during the transfer.
15. Repeat procedure in reverse order for transfer back to the stretcher.

TASK 4-6

Procedure: Logrolling the Patient

Terminal Performance Objective: Provided with a classmate for a patient, two assistant helpers, necessary equipment and supplies, logroll a patient onto the radiographic table. All items on the instructor's checklist must be marked satisfactory or not applicable.

Equipment/Supplies

- Classmate as a simulated patient
- Stretcher
- Radiographic table
- Two classmates to serve as assistant helpers

Performance Guide

1. Wash hands.
2. Ask two other assistants to help. Identify the patient and explain what you plan to do.

3. Position assistants. One assistant should be on the same side of the bed as you are. The other assistant should be at the patient's opposite side to keep patient from falling as he/she rolls. If side rails are available on the stretcher, also secure the side rail.

4. Move the patient as a unit toward you. Place a pillow lengthwise between the patient's legs. Fold his/her arms over his/her chest.

5. Turn the patient to his/her side:

   a. Use a turning sheet that has been previously placed under the patient.
      - Reaching over patient, grasp and roll the turning sheet toward the patient.
      - Position one assistant beside the patient to keep shoulders and hips straight. Second assistant should be positioned to keep thighs and lower legs straight.

   b. If a turning sheet is not in position, the first assistant should position hands on far shoulders and hips. Second assistant positions hands on far thigh and lower leg.

6. At a specified signal, the patient is drawn toward both assistants in a single movement, keeping spine, head, and legs in straight position. Additional pillows are placed behind the patient to maintain the position. A small pillow or folded bath blanket may be permitted under the head and neck. Leave pillow between the legs and position small pillows or folded towels to support the arms until ready for radiographic positioning.

7. Check patient for comfort, alignment, and support.

8. Observe all safety precautions.

9. Use good body alignment and mechanics during the transfer.

TASK 4-7

Procedure: Assisting the Patient with Ambulatory Aid: Cane, Walker, and Crutches

Terminal Performance Objective: Provided with a classmate for a patient, assist the patient with an ambulatory aide to move from the waiting area to the radiographic room and on/off the radiographic table. All items on the instructor's checklist must be marked satisfactory or not applicable.

Equipment/Supplies

- Classmate as a simulated patient

- Cane
- Walker
- Crutches
- Radiographic table

Performance Guide

(The simulated situation should pose such obstacles as doors and hallways similar in width to those found in medical facilities.)

1. Wash hands.
2. Locate and identify the patient.
3. Introduce self and briefly explain purpose of transfer.
4. Assess patient's condition.
5. Assist patient to move from waiting area or reception area to radiography room.
6. Assist patient during disrobing, if applicable.
7. Provide support to the patient's weak side as he/she gets onto and off the radiographic table.
8. Provide for patient safety and comfort needs:
   a. Patient with a cane
   b. Patient with a walker
   c. Patient with crutches

TASK 4-8

Procedure: Transporting the Patient in a Wheelchair

Terminal Performance Objective: Provided with a classmate for a patient, a wheelchair, and a beginning and ending destination, transport a patient in a wheelchair. All items on the instructor's checklist must be marked satisfactory or not applicable.

Equipment/Supplies

- Classmate as a simulated patient
- Wheelchair

Performance Guide

1. Locate and identify the patient.

2. Introduce self and explain procedure.
3. Secure patient's clothing/drapes from possible entanglement.
4. Check to be sure tubes, drainage bottles, catheters, etc., are secure.
5. Release hand brake to unlock wheels.
6. Transport the patient along the right side of the hall.
7. Move through door: (if applicable)
    a. Approach closed doorway backwards.
    b. Use one hand to open door and support door open with body as needed.
    c. Pull chair through backwards.
    d. Turn wheelchair to forward after getting through door.
8. Use elevator: (if applicable)
    a. Secure elevator door.
    b. Pull wheelchair onto elevator backward.
    c. Turn wheelchair around and leave elevator pulling wheelchair backward.
9. Make all turns carefully and smoothly to avoid stress or danger to the patient.
10. When destination is reached set hand brake to lock wheels.

TASK 4-9

Procedure: Transferring the Patient Between Radiographic Table and Wheelchair

Terminal Performance Objective: Provided with a classmate for a patient, wheelchair, radiographic table, and a footstool, transfer the patient between the radiographic table and wheelchair without injury to the patient or damage to equipment. All items on the instructor's checklist must be marked satisfactory or not applicable.

Equipment/Supplies

■ Classmate as a simulated patient
■ Wheelchair
■ Radiographic table
■ Footstool

Performance Guide

1. Wash hands.
2. Locate and identify the patient.

3. Introduce self and explain procedure.
4. Position wheelchair beside table, facing head of table.
5. Set wheel brakes and raise footrests.
6. Assist patient to sitting position on the examination table with legs dangling and remove sheet.
7. Assist patient to standing position on footstool.
8. Assist patient to step down from footstool.
9. Assist patient to pivot and lower body into wheelchair.
10. Reverse procedure to move patient from wheelchair onto examination table.
11. Cover patient with sheet.
12. Ensure patient is comfortable before leaving.
13. Observe all safety precautions.
14. Use good body alignment and mechanics when transferring patient.

TASK 4-10

Procedure: Preparing Patient for Radiographic Examination

Terminal Performance Objective: In a simulated situation, provided with a classmate as a patient, radiographic request, and examination gown, prepare the patient for a radiographic examination. All items on the instructor's checklist must be rated acceptable or not applicable.

Equipment/Supplies

- Classmate as a simulated patient
- Prepare patient situations on 3″ × 5″ card so that the simulated patient will be required to present specific patient situations.
- Examination room or privacy screen.
- Radiographic request—request should be for a specific body area that will require the student to request that the patient disrobe. In practice situation, student should be provided with situations that are reality-based—e.g., patient with mastectomy who requires assistance in removing clothing.
- Examination gown.

Performance Guide

1. Review radiographic request.
2. Locate and identify patient.

Key Point: In some medical facilities, the patient may be waiting in the reception room. To avoid miscommunication, use a clear, articulate voice when saying the patient's name. Always ask the patient his/her name. Do not say to a patient, "Are you Mr(s). Smith?" He/she may misunderstand and nod or confirm to the wrong identity.

3. Introduce self and explain procedure.
4. Assess patient's physical ability.
   Key Point: Never leave a patient unattended or alone to disrobe if he/she is unstable or seems confused. *Never* leave young children unattended.
5. Give the patient instructions to disrobe and don examination gown.
   Key Point: Be very specific as to what articles of clothing should be removed. Be specific regarding undergarments, jewelry, or any opaque objects.
   a. Assist patient in removing clothing.
   b. Explain how to put on examination gown.
   c. Take care of patient's valuables.

TASK 4-11

Procedure: Taking Temperature by Mercury and Electronic Thermometers

Terminal Performance Objective: Provided with a classmate for a patient, necessary equipment, and supplies, take and record the patient's oral temperature. Methods of measurement will be a mercury thermometer and an electronic thermometer. All items on the instructor's checklist must be rated satisfactory or not applicable.

Equipment/Supplies

■ Classmate as a simulated patient
■ Sterilization supplies if thermometers are not disposable
■ Oral, glass tube thermometer with elongated tip
■ Electronic thermometer with disposable sheath covers
■ Blunt tip (short rounded) rectal thermometer (to be used for demonstration only).

Performance Guide

1. Wash hands.

2. Locate and identify the patient.
3. Introduce self and explain procedure to the patient.
4. *Mercury Thermometer:* Pick up thermometer and wipe; if necessary, rinse off antiseptic solution in cool water.

    or

    Electronic Thermometer: Apply sterile protective disposable sheath cover to electronic thermometer.
5. Shake mercury down to 96°F or 36.5°C; or set electronic digital scale.
6. Appropriately insert thermometer.
7. Leave thermometer in place the required amount of time, or until buzzer signals for electronic thermometer.
8. Remove and read scale.
9. Clean thermometer or discard sheath.
10. Replace thermometer in holder.
11. Record patient's temperature.

TASK 4-12

Procedure: Counting the Radial Pulse and Respiratory Rate

Terminal Performance Objective: Provided with a classmate for a patient, take and record the patient's radial pulse and respiratory rate. All items on the instructor's checklist must be marked acceptable or not applicable.

Equipment/Supplies

- Classmate as a simulated patient
- Watch with second hand

Performance Guide

1. Wash hands.
2. Locate and identify patient.
3. Place patient in a comfortable position. The palm of the hand should be down and the arm should rest across the patient's chest.
4. Locate the pulse on the thumb side of the wrist with the tips of your first three fingers. Do not use your thumb since it contains a pulse that may be confused with the patient's pulse.

5. When the pulse is felt, exert slight pressure. Use second hand of watch and count for one minute.
6. When the pulse rate has been counted, leave the fingers on the radial pulse and start counting the number of times the chest rises and falls during one minute.
7. Note depth and regularity of respirations.
8. Record the pulse rate, time, rhythm, and the regularity and depth of respirations.

TASK 4-13

Procedure: Taking Blood Pressure

Terminal Performance Objective: Provided with a classmate for a patient and necessary equipment and supplies, take and record the patient's blood pressure. All items on the instructor's checklist must be marked acceptable or not applicable.

Equipment/Supplies

- Classmate as a simulated patient
- Stethoscope
- Blood pressure cuff
- Sphygmomanometer (mercury or aneroid)

Performance Guide

1. Wash hands.
2. Locate and identify the patient.
3. Assemble the equipment needed: sphygmomanometer and stethoscope. (Clean stethoscope earpieces and bell with antiseptic solution.)
4. Place the patient's arm palm-upward, supported on bed or table.
5. Roll sleeve of patient's gown up about five inches above elbow. Be sure it is not tight on the arm.
6. Apply cuff smoothly and evenly one to one-and-one-half inches above the elbow. The center of the rubber bladder should be directly over the brachial artery. The brachial artery is located on the inside of the arm (medial aspect) just inside the elbow. If the cuff is marked with an arrow, place cuff so that the arrow points over the brachial artery.
7. Tuck ends of cuff and hook to secure closure. Be sure cuff is secure but not too tight. Check by slipping two fingers between cuff and patient's arm.

8. Locate the radial artery and palpate it as you:
    a. Close valve attached to hand pump (air bulb) by turning it clockwise.
    b. Quickly inflate cuff until the gauge registers 50 mm Hg.
    c. Continue to inflate cuff in 10-mm-Hg increments until radial pulse cannot be felt. This pressure indicates the palpated systolic pressure. Note the pressure.
    d. Quickly deflate cuff by turning the close valve counterclockwise.
9. Ask the patient to raise the arm and flex fingers.
10. Locate the brachial artery with the fingers.
11. Place earpieces in ears. Place bell of stethoscope directly over the artery.
12. Close valve and reinflate cuff quickly until gauge registers 30 mm above palpated systolic pressure.
13. Listen carefully as you open valve of pump by turning counterclockwise.
14. Let air escape slowly (between 1–3 mm per second) until first heart sound is heard. Note reading on manometer at top of meniscus as the systolic pressure.
15. Continue to release the air pressure slowly until there is an abrupt change of the sound from very loud to a soft muffled sound. The reading at which this change is heard is the diastolic pressure. In some facilities, the last sound heard is taken as the diastolic pressure.
16. Rapidly deflate cuff and remove, expel air from the cuff, and replace apparatus. Clean earpieces and bell of stethoscope with antiseptic solution.
    Note: If repeat procedure is necessary, wait at least one minute.
    a. As patient to raise arm and flex fingers.
    b. Repeat procedure.
17. Remember to wash your hands, report completion of task, and document date, time, systolic and diastolic readings as an improper fraction, patient's reaction, and site of reading if other than the brachial artery.

TASK 7-1

Procedure: Cleaning Radiographic Facilities and Equipment

Terminal Performance Objective: Given a radiographic room, clean the facilities and equipment. Area must be clean and free of dust.

Equipment/Supplies

- Radiographic equipment (table, tube stand console)
- Cleaning solutions

- Cleaning cloths
- Gloves (if needed to protect hands)

Performance Guide

1. Place dampened or wet items, such as dressings and bandages, in waterproof bags and close bags tightly before discarding.
2. Dust mechanical parts of the X-ray machine with a clean, damp (not wet) cloth.
3. Clean table with a disinfectant beginning with the least dirty to the most dirty area.
4. Clean metal parts with benzine or a solution specified by the hospital procedure manual.
5. Polish metal parts.
6. Clean overhead parts (X-ray tube and other parts that conduct electricity) with alcohol or a clean, dry cloth.
   CAUTION: Never use water to clean electrical parts.
   Note: Clean cones, compression devices, and other accessories daily.
7. Dissolve adhesive-tape residue from cassettes with benzine, then wash with alcohol or warm soapy water.
8. Put fresh linen on table and pillow.
   Note: Make sure that rags and mops are disinfected and dried before reuse.

TASK 7-2

Procedure: Operating Radiographic Tables and Consoles

Terminal Performance Objective: Provided with a classmate for a patient and necessary equipment and supplies, perform the functions listed in the performance guide.

Equipment/Supplies

- Buckey tray
- Cassettes
- Student (to act as patient)
- Tissue caliper

Performance Guide

Each student will

1. Properly place various sizes of cassettes in the bucky tray.
2. Properly align the CR with the table top and with the film (cassette) in the bucky tray.
3. Raise and lower the table with a patient (another student) on the table.
4. Use a caliper to measure various parts of another student. Use supine and standing positions.

TASK 9-1

Procedure: Testing Safelight Performance

Terminal Performance Objective: Given a cassette, radiographic film, radiographic equipment, and a film processor, determine whether the safelight is fogging the film. All items on the instructor's checklist must be rated satisfactory or not applicable.

Equipment/Supplies

- Cassette
- Radiographic film (exposed)
- Radiographic equipment (energized)
- Film processor
- Safelight illuminator

Performance Guide

1. Select two cassettes loaded with film.
2. Expose each to a very minimal X-ray exposure (about 10.0 mAs, 60 kv, 40″ SID).
   Note: Both cassettes must receive exactly the same exposure.
3. Remove the film from one cassette under conditions that normally exist in the darkroom and process the film.
4. Turn off safelight(s) and remove the film from the remaining cassette.
   Note: This step must be accomplished in total darkness.
5. Process the film.
6. Check the film for differences in density by placing side by side on the same viewbox.

TASK 9-2

Procedure: Maintaining Master Card File or Computer System

Terminal Performance Objective: Provided with a master card file system or a computer terminal, a listing of examinations performed, and necessary patient data, enter the information on the card file or computer file. Each entry must include the patient's name, identification number, age, birth date, examination name, date, X-ray file number, and the physician's and operator's names. All items on the instructor's checklist must be marked satisfactory or not applicable.

Equipment/Supplies

- Pen/pencil
- Master cards or computer system information
- Master card files or computer file
- Patient's chart
- Daily examination record

Performance Guide

1. Obtain patient's updated medical file.
2. Locate patient's master card (file on computer).
   Note: If no master card or computer file exists, the operator must create one. (See step 3 for required information.)
3. Remove master card and record update information or record updated information in computer file:
   a. patient's name and age/birth date
   b. patient's identification number
   c. examination name and date
   d. X-ray file number
   e. physician's name
   f. operator's name
4. Verify that update information is correct.
5. Place master card in correct location according to filing system used or store computer information properly.

TASK 9-3

Procedure: Indexing and Filing Radiographs

Terminal Performance Objective: Given radiographs and film folders, index and file them according to the established filing system. All items must be filed in the patient's folder according to the established filing system. All items on the instructor's checklist must be marked satisfactory or not applicable.

Equipment/Supplies

- Radiographic requests
- Radiographs
- Filing/index system
- Storage receptacle
- Interpretation records

Performance Guide

1. Determine the system of filing:
   a. numerical
   b. alphabetical
   c. disease code index
   d. color code
2. Check for previous radiographs or examinations.
3. Index the folder(s) by writing identifying information on the film folders.
   a. patient name
   b. examination
   c. patient number
   d. date
   e. physician
4. Place radiograph(s) and folder(s) in the diagnostic reading area.
5. After diagnostic interpretation, place radiographs in corresponding film folder(s).
6. File the folder(s).

TASK 9-4

Procedure: Processing Loans of Radiographs

Terminal Performance Objective: Given a request for a loan of radiographs, process the radiographs for loan. All information must be recorded on the mailing folder and the patient's permanent folder without error. All items on the instructor's checklist must be marked satisfactory or not applicable.

Equipment/Supplies

- Loan request
- Radiographs
- Master card file system
- Requested radiographs

Performance Guide

1. Retrieve film to be loaned; determine return due date.
2. Place duplicates of the radiographs in a loan folder.
3. Write patient's name, radiographic number, and physician's name on loan folder.
4. Address folder; include return address.
5. Record the following: date, to whom films were loaned (complete address), and number and size of films sent. Also note the return due date on patient's permanent folder and in the patient's medical file, where applicable.

TASK 9-5

Procedure: Loading and Unloading a Cassette

Terminal Performance Objective: Provided with a cassette, film, and a darkroom environment, load and unload the cassette. The film must not be fogged nor contain artifacts. The intensifying screen must be free of damage. All items on the instructor's checklist must be marked satisfactory or not applicable.

Equipment/Supplies

- Cassette (authors suggest providing student practice with the following: hinge cassette and two pressure bar cassettes)

- X-ray film
- Darkroom environment

Performance Guide

1. Place cassette, with exposed film on work area.
2. Close darkroom door, turn off white lights.
3. Turn on safelight.
4. Open film holder. (See note under equipment and supplies regarding practice with a variety of film holders.)
5. Tip front of cassette.
   Note: This tipping allows the film to fall free of the cassette borders.
6. Grasp film gently at an edge or corner.
7. Lift film out of film holder.
8. Grasp film on corner opposite of side of film being lifted. (This avoids a kink mark in the film.)
9. Insert film into printer. (The next step, processing the film, should be used only if student is ready for this step.)

Reloading a cassette:

10. Open film bin or storage container.
11. Grasp unexposed film with thumb and forefinger.
12. Lift out of film box/bin.
13. Grasp bottom edge with thumb and forefinger of other hand.
14. Load cassette using both hands.
15. Close or secure cassette.
16. Place loaded film holder with other unexposed cassettes.
17. Check to determine if film bin is closed or film safely covered.
18. Turn on white lights.
19. Open door and exit.

TASK 9-6

Procedure: Cleaning Intensifying Screens

Terminal Performance Objective: Given a cassette, screen cleaner, and a cleaning cloth, clean the intensifying screen. Screen must not be nicked, scratched, or chipped while being cleaned, and must be free of smudges and foreign particles. All items on the instructor's checklist must be marked satisfactory or not applicable.

Equipment/Supplies

■ Cassette
■ Screen cleaner (use commercial brand recommended by screen manufacturer)
■ Soft, lint-free cloth

Performance Guide

1. Turn off white lights and turn on safelight.
2. Unload cassette in darkroom (follow directions for handling film). Put unexposed film in film bin or storage container. Secure film bin from light exposure.
3. Turn white lights on.
4. Check screens for dust or foreign materials.
5. Wipe screens with screen cleaner.
   a. Pour cleaner onto soft cloth. *Do not pour solution on screens.*
   b. Rub gently in circular direction. Overlap strokes.
   c. Care must be taken not to nick, scratch, or chip the screens.
6. Dry screen with lint-free cloth.
7. Stand the half-opened cassette on its side for about one-half hour in a dust-free room for further drying. If the cassette screen has been numbered for future film identification matching, these numbers may require remarking after cleaning.* Check to determine that the inside cassette number matches the number on the outside of the cassette.
8. Reload cassette with unexposed film.
9. Record cassette number, date cleaned, and any significant findings.
10. If screen appears damaged, report to appropriate supervisor.

Note: If unwanted shadows or artifacts appear on the finished radiograph, having a number on the screen and on the outside of the cassette will help to quickly locate the cassette in question.

TASK 9-7

Procedure: Testing Cassette for Screen-Film Contact (See Figure 9-14.)

Terminal Performance Objective: Given a cassette, radiographic film, a wire mesh or screen, radiographic equipment and processor, perform a screen-film contact test. Determine whether the cassette has proper screen-film contact. All items on the instructor's checklist must be marked satisfactory or not applicable.

Equipment/Supplies

- Cassette(s)
- Wire mesh or screen (sized to cover entire front of the cassette being tested)
- Radiographic equipment (energized)
- Radiographic processor
- Radiographic film

Performance Guide

1. Assemble supplies and cassettes in radiographic room.
2. Place wire mesh or screen over cassette. Cassette should be positioned under X-ray beam.
3. Set exposure factors (usually 50 kvp, 1/20 second, 50 mA, 40 in SID).
4. Make exposure.
5. Process film.
6. Check radiograph for areas of blurring.*
7. Record findings. A log should be maintained that contains the number of the cassette tested, the date, and the results. Any areas of blurring should be reported to supervisor.
8. Straighten the work area.

Note: It is easier to stand five to six feet back from the viewing illuminator. At this distance, blurred areas will stand out as areas of darker density. If a blurred area appears, it indicates that the screen is warped. The cassette must be repaired or discarded. Today, most manufacturers recommend that the cassette be discarded.

TASK 9-8

Procedure: Processing Film by Manual Method (See Figure 9-19)

Terminal Performance Objective: Provided with manual processing tanks, thermometer, stir stick, timer, processing hanger, a darkroom environment, and a film holder containing exposed film, process the film in manual processing tanks. The film must be free of artifacts and must not be fogged. All items on the instructor's checklist must be marked satisfactory or not applicable.

Equipment/Supplies

- Cassette containing exposed film

- ■ Manual processing tanks
- ■ Thermometer
- ■ Stir sticks (one for developer and one for fixer)
- ■ Timer
- ■ Darkroom environment

Performance Guide

1. Assemble all necessary supplies.
2. Close darkroom door and secure.
3. Stir developer solution.
   - ■ Check water temperature using thermometer.
   - ■ Determine development and fixation time.
   - ■ Stir solutions.
   - ■ Determine if chemical level and activity is sufficient for processing.
4. Mix stop bath solution, if available. (Always use clean stir stick.)
5. Mix fixer solution.
6. Read chemical thermometer.*
7. Determine development time.*
8. Determine fixation time.*
9. Set processing timer, but do not start.
10. Turn off white lights and turn on safelight.
11. Unload cassette.
12. Load wire hanger.
13. Immerse film in developer solution and start the timer.
14. Agitate film gently to dislodge air bubbles.
15. Remove film from developer when timer goes off. (Do not drain in tank.)
16. Rinse film in wash bath for thirty seconds. Allow excess water to drain off.
17. Immerse film in fixer solution and start the timer.
18. Agitate film gently to dislodge air bubbles.
19. Remove film from solution when timer goes off.
20. Rinse film in final wash for twenty to thirty minutes, depending upon the rate of water exchange (recommended rate of water exchange is eight times per hour).
21. Suspend hanger in dryer or drip rack.
22. Clip the corners of the dry radiograph. This prevents snagging on other films.
23. Straighten work area. Reload film holder in darkroom environment.

Note: Determine by using manufacturer's suggested time/temperature guidelines. (See Figure 9-20.)

TASK 9-9

Procedure: Processing Film by Automatic Method

Terminal Performance Objective: Provided with an automatic processor, a darkroom environment, and a cassette containing exposed film, process the film using the automatic processor. The film must be free of artifacts and must not be fogged. All items on the instructor's checklist must be marked satisfactory or not applicable.

Equipment/Supplies

- Exposed radiograph in cassette
- Safelight illumination
- Automatic processor
- Darkroom environment

Performance Guide

1. Enter darkroom, turn off white light.
2. Check for white-light leaks.
3. Turn on safelight illuminator.
4. Open cassette.
5. Remove film and place on feed tray according to manufacturer's recommendations.
   CAUTION: Do not touch face of film. Grasp film by edges.
6. Push film forward until it is caught by rollers.
   Note: Bell will ring or a dimly lit flasher light will flash to indicate that the film is completely in the processor and replenishment has stopped.
7. Reload cassette.
8. Secure door on film bin and turn on white lights.
9. Open door and exit.
10. Retrieve processed film when it emerges from processor.

Index